The 1889-1890 Flu Pandemic: The History of the 19th Century's Last Major Global Outbreak

By Charles River Editors

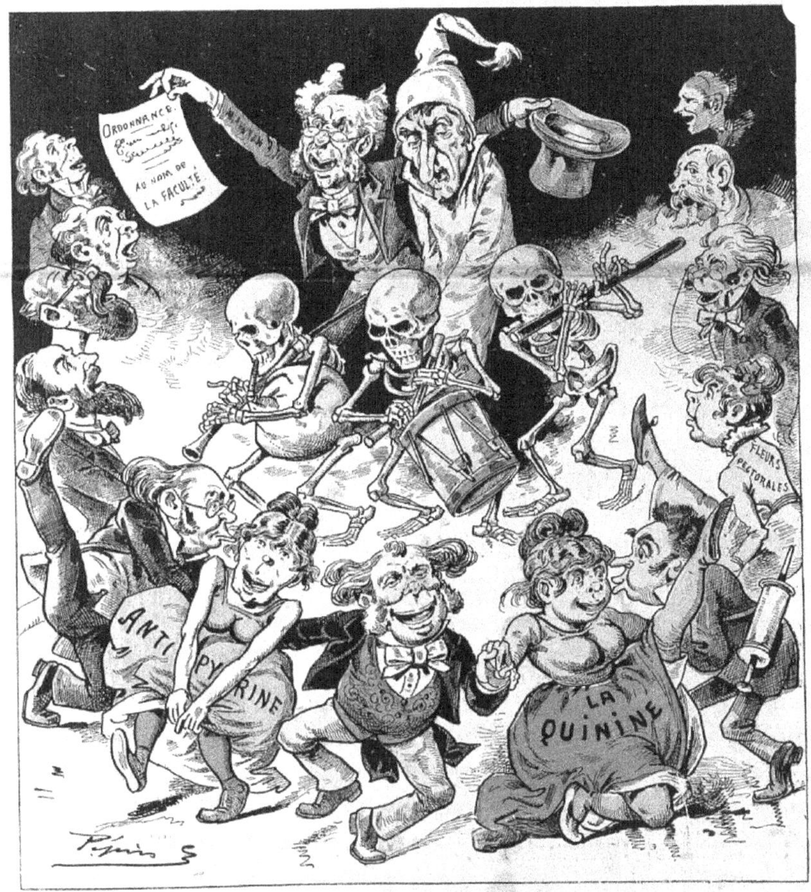

La Ronde des Médecins et des Potards.

A January 1890 cartoon from *Le Grelot* depicting a flu victim being hassled by a crowd of doctors, musicians, and drug sellers

Introduction

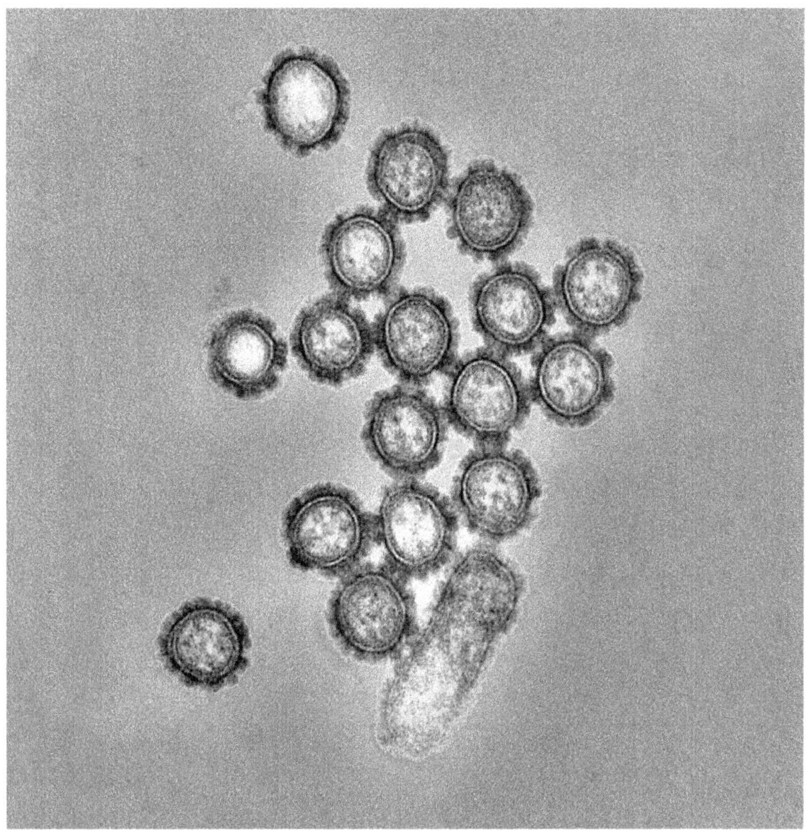

An electron micrograph of the virus

Plague and pestilence have both fascinated and terrified humanity from the very beginning. Societies and individuals have struggled to make sense of them, and more importantly they've often struggled to avoid them. Before the scientific age, people had no knowledge of the microbiological agents – unseen bacteria and viruses – which afflicted them, and thus the maladies were often ascribed to wrathful supernatural forces. Even when advances in knowledge posited natural causes for epidemics and pandemics, medicine struggled to deal with them, and for hundreds of years religion continued to work hand-in-hand with medicine.

Inevitably, that meant physicians tried a variety of practices to cure the sick, and many of them seem quite odd by modern standards. By the time Rome was on the rise, physicians understood that contagions arose and spread, but according to Galen, Hippocrates, and other Greco-Roman authorities, pestilence was caused by *miasma*, foul air produced by the decomposition of organic matter. Though modern scientists have since been able to disprove this, on the face of it there was some logic to the idea. Physicians and philosophers (they were very often the same, Galen being an example) noticed that disease arose in areas of poor sanitation, where filth and rotting matter was prevalent and not disposed of, and the basic measures to prevent disease – waste removal, provision of clean food and water and quarantining - would have been obvious to them.

The scenting of miasmic air with incense and other unguents to expel the foulness would also have thus made sense, though people now know that can't stop the spread of a disease.

It was only in the mid-19th century that scientists established a definitive link between viruses and bacteria and disease, and this allowed the development of vaccines to prevent the spread of killers such as smallpox, typhus, and diphtheria. In the early 20th century, the development of antibiotics helped immensely, but as the Spanish flu of 1918 and the recent Coronavirus demonstrated, people have not succeeded in conquering all infectious diseases. In fact, it was not until World War II that most of the pestilences that have afflicted people in the past could be effectively prevented, and the fear of contagion remains strong.

One of these plagues is influenza, a disease now regarded almost with contempt as being a minimal threat to life, but it is actually one of the greatest killers of modern times, taking up to 650,000 lives every year.[1] It may come as a surprise for many to learn that there is no single vaccine for the flu - there are vaccines for the strains that presently exist, but new strains evolve every year, so vaccines must be constantly developed. Influenza remains one of the greatest threats to public health and challenges to the medical profession.

The first known influenza pandemic may have occurred in China in 6000 BCE,[2] and the renowned Greek physician Hippocrates described the symptoms of influenza around 600 BCE.[3] The first well-documented pandemic, however, occurred in 1580. It originated in East Asia, spread through Central Asia and the Russian Empire, and then on to Europe. In Rome, about 8,000 people perished and some settlements in Spain disappeared entirely.[4] Europeans brought it to the Americas in the 16th century, where it may contributed to decimating the indigenous populations.[5] After that, flu epidemics hit Europe sporadically for more than 200 years, with that of 1830–33 being one of the worst, when about 25% of 135 million Europeans were infected.

Therefore, when an outbreak of flu occurred in the Central Asian city of Bukhara in 1889, it could not have excited any great concern. Certainly, some nearby communities may have anxiously braced themselves, but epidemics had occurred before and Europe had survived. Besides, then – as now – influenza was a disease that affected mostly the elderly and ill. But Europe – and the world – had changed profoundly in recent times. Its states had been industrializing, experimenting with new methods of communication, transportation, and trade, and these very innovations would be the means of spreading the flu, not just through Europe, but across the entire world. For the first time in its history, the world faced a pestilence that would

---

[1] "Up to 650,000 people die of respiratory diseases linked to seasonal flu each year". World Health Organization *(WHO)* (Press release). 14 December 2017.

[2] Mordini E, Green M, eds. (2013). *Internet-Based Intelligence in Public Health Emergencies: Early Detection and Response in Disease Outbreak Crises*. IOS Press. p. 67.

[3] Martin PM, Martin-Granel E (June 2006). "2,500-year evolution of the term epidemic". *Emerging Infectious Diseases*. **12** (6): 976–80.

[4] Potter CW (October 2001). "A history of influenza". *Journal of Applied Microbiology*. **91** (4): 572–79.

[5] Guerra F (1988). "The earliest American epidemic. The influenza of 1493". *Social Science History*. **12** (3): 305–25.

cross every geographical barrier, even the oceans. This meant it would not be an epidemic but a pandemic, embracing the entire globe in its deadly grip.

The 1889-1890 Flu Pandemic: The History of the 19th Century's Last Major Global Outbreak looks at how the pandemic started, what was done to fight the virus, and its impact on the world. Along with pictures depicting important people, places, and events, you will learn about the outbreak like never before.

The Outbreak

The Emirate of Bukhara was founded in 1785 and occupied the territory between the Amu Darya and Syr Darya Rivers in Transoxania in Central Asia, thus covering an area a little larger than the present United Kingdom. Today its former dominions are divided between Uzbekistan and Tajikistan, and its chief cities were Bukhara, the capital, and Samarkand, the former capital of the old Timurid Empire. The emirate was the last remnant of the Mongol Empire that had at one time ruled the greater part of Asia, the Middle East and Russia, and although its emir did not claim blood descent from Genghis Khan, he nevertheless gloried in his Mongol heritage.

At the time, the Russian Empire was vigorously pursuing a policy of territorial expansion in Asia, and one by one the weaker Muslim states in the Caucasus and Central Asia succumbed to its arms. In February 1866, it was Bukhara's turn, and after a two-year war, Emir Muzaffar al-Din bin Nasr-Allah surrendered upon the understanding that he would remain as ruler but be subordinate to the Russian tsars.

The Bukharan emirate was one of the more prosperous of the Central Asian states thanks to its location along the trade route between China and the Middle East, and thus it depended heavily on trade. The Trans-Caspian Railway, begun by the imperial Russian government to accommodate its Asian conquests, also reached Bukhara in 1888, enhancing the wealth of both Russian and Bukharan merchants. By then, Bukhara was also one of the most urbanized of the Russian protectorates, with up to 14% of the population living in towns and cities.[6]

The emir ruled as an autocrat according to traditional Islamic law and tradition, and despite encouraging some Western reforms, the Russian Empire was content to leave him to rule as he wished. But Bukhara was not content to leave Russia undisturbed, as the events of 1889 were to prove. In May of that year influenza broke out in the emirate's capital, and there was nothing peculiar in that since pestilences frequently afflicted Central Asia and had done so for millennia. Indeed, plagues were continuing to ravage the developed nations of Europe and the Americas at the time, and just 30 years earlier, a million people had died of cholera in Russia alone. It is estimated that up to two-thirds of Bokhara's population perished,[7] and as tragic as that was, it would not normally have presaged anything worse at the time - Bukhara was geographically isolated, even from the rest of the emirate, owing to mountains, rivers, and deserts, and the pestilence would probably have not spread significantly if it had not been for the Trans-Caspian Railway.

Indeed, the desire to link Central Asia with the rest of the world unwittingly let the epidemic

[6] Seymour Becker (2004), *Russia's Protectorates in Central Asia: Bukhara and Khiva 1865–1924*, Routledge, p.5.

[7] George C. Kohn (2007), *Encyclopedia of Plague and Pestilence: From Ancient Times to the Present*, Infobase Publishing p.21.

loose. By August, the flu was beginning to abate in Bukhara, but by then it had taken hold in Samarkand, and in October it reached the Siberian city of Tomsk, about 3,200 kilometers to the northeast. Tomsk was on a trade route from Moscow to China, but it was a road, not a railway (work on the Trans-Siberian Railway did not begin until 1891), which slowed down the spread of the epidemic in that direction. Nevertheless, it reached Krasnovodsk (modern Turkmenbasy) on the Caspian Sea, the westernmost station of the Trans-Caspian, and from there the disease infected the Volga trade routes, reaching Moscow and St. Petersburg at about the same time. In the process, the disease spread to Constantinople, the capital of the Ottoman Empire.

The epidemic struck St Petersburg particularly hard, with as many as 180,000 people, including the tsar, incapacitated. The city had a little less than a million inhabitants at the time, and it was reported that the malady struck suddenly, causing very high temperatures, swollen hands, face rashes, and unbearable body aches. The only mercy was that these afflictions usually lasted no more than six days and then disappeared as quickly as they had come.[8]

In mid-November 1889, the epidemic had reached Kiev, and a month later it struck the Lake Baikal region in southern Siberia. It was now on the verge of invading China. By July of the following year, all of Siberia and Sakhalin Island were infected.

The strain or subtype of the influenza virus was possibly influenza A virus subtype H2N2 (A/H2N2), though studies to this day remain inconclusive.[9] Symptoms of influenza include fever, coughing, sore throat, running nose, fatigue, muscle pain and headache, and severe cases can produce shortness of breath, chest pain, confusion, vomiting and dehydration. Most people today recover from the flu, with a small minority dying of pneumonia, sepsis (blood poisoning), or complications due to preexisting conditions.[10] However, in the 19th century the general standard of health and medical knowledge was much lower than it is today. In early 19th century Britain the average life expectancy was still only forty,[11] and even by the beginning of the 20th century the world average was just 31.[12] In pre-industrial states such as Bukhara, living

---

8

Bogumiła Kempińska-Mirosławska and Agnieszka WoŸniak-Kosek, "The influenza epidemic of 1889–90 in selected European cities – a picture based on the reports of two Poznań daily newspapers from the second half of the 19th century", US National Library of Medicine https://www.ncbi.nlm.nih.gov/pmc/articles/PMC3867475/#__sec7title.

[9] Hilleman, Maurice R. (2002). "Realities and enigmas of human viral influenza: pathogenesis, epidemiology and control". *Vaccine*. **20** (25–26): 3068–3087.

[10] Sarah Klein, "Why Do Some People Die From the Flu?" *Health.com* January 24 2019 https://www.health.com/condition/cold-flu-sinus/how-do-you-die-from-flu.

[11] Galor, Oded; Moav, Omer (2005). "Natural Selection and the Evolution of Life Expectancy" (PDF). *Brown University Working Paper*. Retrieved November 4, 2010.

[12] Prentice, Thomson. "Health, history and hard choices: Funding dilemmas in a fast-changing world" (PDF). *World*

conditions would have been harsh and challenging.

For nearly 2,000 years, it was believed pestilence was caused by *miasma*, foul air produced by the decomposition of organic matter. Though modern scientists have since been able to disprove this, on the face of it there was some logic to the idea. Physicians and philosophers (they were very often the same, Galen being an example) noticed that disease arose in areas of poor sanitation, where filth and rotting matter was prevalent and not disposed of, and the basic measures to prevent disease – waste removal, provision of clean food and water and quarantining - would have been obvious to them. The scenting of miasmic air with incense and other unguents to expel the foulness would also have thus made sense, though people now know that can't stop the spread of a disease.

Ancient physicians at the time believed that *miasma* was not the direct cause of disease but rather a catalyst. Maladies were caused by an imbalance of what Galen called the four humors. According to him (and Hippocrates before him), the body contained four kinds of fluids: black bile, yellow bile, blood, and phlegm. These corresponded to the four elements of which the entire universe was composed: earth, fire, water, and air. Black bile was tied to earth, yellow bile to fire, blood to air, and phlegm to water. It was believed that the balance of the humors in the body not only determined an individual's health, but their behavior and temperament as well. A melancholic (from *melanos*, the word for "black") disposition was caused by an excess of black bile. Yellow bile made a person fiery or choleric (from *khole*, the word for bile), while a phlegmatic (from *phlegma*, body moisture) temperament denoted a surplus of phlegm. The most desirable temperament was the sanguine (*sanguis*, blood), which exhibited happiness, calm and enthusiasm. The ancient Romans thought *miasma* caused an imbalance in these fluids, and disease resulted. For the ancient physician, as indeed for all physicians for the next 1,500 years or so, illness was not the direct result of external agents.

The theory of the four humors was based on philosophy rather than what today would be called science. It might seem easy to ridicule the idea in hindsight, but the ancient philosophers and doctors did not and could not possess the elementary scientific knowledge that medical practitioners have today, so humorism can be seen as an honest attempt to make sense of the human body and its malignancies.

The High Middle Ages had seen a rise in Western Europe's population in previous centuries, but these gains were almost entirely erased as the plague spread rapidly across all of Europe from 1346-1353. With a medieval understanding of medicine, diagnosis, and illness, nobody understood what caused Black Death or how to truly treat it. As a result, many religious people assumed it was divine retribution, while superstitious and suspicious citizens saw a nefarious human plot involved and persecuted certain minority groups among them.

Health Organization: Global Health Histories. Retrieved November 4, 2010.

Though it is now widely believed that rats and fleas spread the disease by carrying the bubonic plague westward along well-established trade routes, and there are now vaccines to prevent the spread of the plague, the Black Death gruesomely killed upwards of 100 million people, with helpless chroniclers graphically describing the various stages of the disease. It took Europe decades for its population to bounce back, and similar plagues would affect various parts of the world for the next several centuries, but advances in medical technology have since allowed researchers to read various medieval accounts of the Black Death in order to understand the various strains of the disease.

Thus, the idea that infectious diseases were caused by microscopic organisms and not by corrupted air named *miasma* was relatively new in 1889, having been demonstrated by Louis Pasteur, Robert Koch, and other scientists. Little was known scientifically about influenza, and it would not be identified as a virus until 1933.[13] By 1889, there were vaccines for cholera and rabies, but influenza vaccines were not produced until 1942.[14]

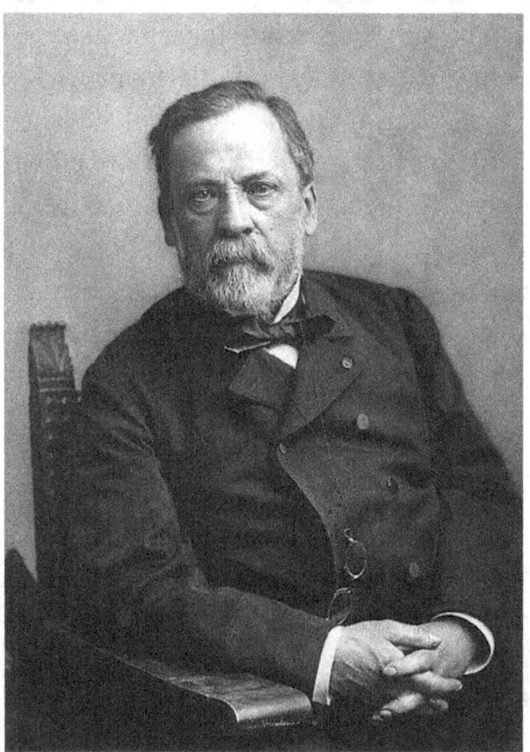

Pasteur

The Russian Empire was ill-prepared to deal with the outbreak when it came, as conditions there were among the most unsanitary in Europe. At the time, the average life expectancy in Russia was 40, a third of newborns died,[15] and contagions such as cholera, typhoid fever and

---

[13] "Influenza Historic Timeline", *Centers for Disease Control and Prevention* January 30 2019
https://www.cdc.gov/flu/pandemic-resources/pandemic-timeline-1930-and-beyond.htm.
[14] Ibid.

smallpox were widespread. There was no organized public healthcare, and the great majority of the population was impoverished, having only been emancipated from serfdom in 1861. In fact, emancipation had only worsened people's lots in life, as peasants were still tied to the land of their masters in order to financially recompense them for their freedom. The tsar, Alexander III, who had fallen ill of the flu himself but recovered, turned his back on reform safter the assassination of his father, Alexander II (r. 1855–1881), and he did little to improve the lot of his subjects. The masses relied on herbal remedies, religion, sorcery and quackery, while only the aristocracy and landed gentry had access to organized medicine.

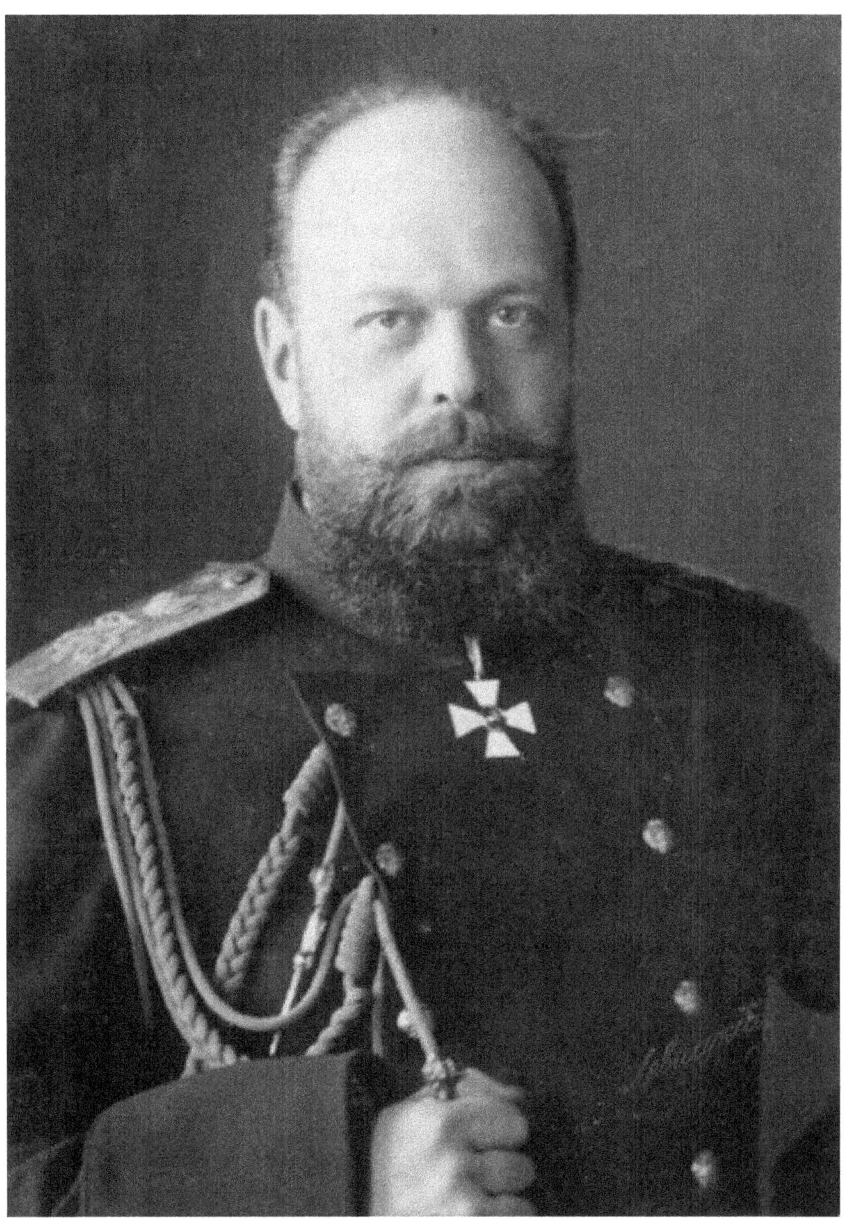

---

[15] Vladimir A. Reshetnikov , Natalia V. Ekkert , Lorenzo Capasso , Evgeny V. Arsentyev , Maria S. Mikerova , Irina I. Yakushina, "The history of public healthcare in Russia", Medicina Historica 2019; Vol. 3, N. 1: 16–24.

The irony of the situation was that the Russian government was attempting to reform, at least with regard to the economy and the military, in order to compete with the other major powers of Europe, and these reforms exacerbated the epidemic. The government constructed railways to facilitate trade and the transportation of goods and troops across the vast empire, and a modern merchant navy traversed the Baltic Sea, Atlantic Ocean, Black Sea, and the Mediterranean. It was inevitable then that a disease originating in Russia would spill out into Europe, the Middle East, and Asia. From those places, it could reach every corner of the globe.

The Pandemic

Once the pestilence swept up the Volga from the Caspian to St Petersburg, it all but ensured the first nations outside Russia to be infected were those that were immediately linked by the Baltic trade routes. In early November of 1889, an outbreak occurred in an artillery corps stationed at Vaxholm, an island about 20 kilometers northeast of Stockholm in the Kingdom of Sweden. From there it spread to Stockholm, and within eight weeks it had infected 60% of the population. Sweden was not a heavily urbanized country, but it was rapidly industrializing, and the flu followed the railways and the coasts, linked by shipping, where most people lived. Rural areas bore the brunt of the mortality, probably on account of the poor living conditions of the peasantry.

From Sweden the influenza passed swiftly into Norway, which shared the same monarch with Sweden at the time, followed by the Kingdom of Denmark. By December 1889, Central Europe, which was primarily under the control of Germany and the Austro-Hungarian Empire, was infected. For centuries Germany had been a nebulous collection of principalities and city-states, but following the defeat of France in the Franco-Prussian War (1870–1871), it had been united into a single empire under the domination of Prussia. In the wake of that union, the new German Empire was rapidly becoming the most industrialized state in continental Europe, and in particular, German unification greatly stimulated the growth of railways. At the time of the empire's inception in 1871, its domains already had 21,000 kilometers of railroad and a fleet of merchant vessels up and down the Rhine. The contagion could therefore spread to every part of Germany in a matter of days.

The disease first appeared in Poznan in South Prussia (now part of Poland). On December 12, newspapers reported that 600 workers contracted influenza in Berlin and Spandau, but by the next day the burden of infection was proving too much for Berlin physicians, suggesting that

Bogumiła Kempińska-Mirosławska et alii.

initial reports had been inaccurate. Just a few days later, influenza cases reached 150,000 (the population of Berlin was just 1.5 million) and had affected every occupation in the city, including the medical profession.[16] Universities suspended lectures, government officials could not carry out their functions, and even essential services such as the fire brigade were crippled. In cities throughout Germany, schools were controversially closed, despite the fact a number of experts claimed that influenza was not as great a threat to children as to adults. Coal mines were also closed, resulting in a temporary drop in the German economy.

It is estimated that at least half of the population in Berlin, including young children, contracted the disease.[17] Johanna Friederike, Princess of Bismarck and wife of Chancellor Otto von Bismarck, suffered from it severely but did not die. The pestilence even made it into the imperial household, and both the former Emperor Wilhelm I (r. 1871–1888) and his wife Augusta fell sick. Wilhelm I survived, but his empress succumbed on January 7, 1890 of pneumonia. Her grandson, Emperor Wilhelm II (r. 1888–1918), was grief-stricken.

[17] Ibid.

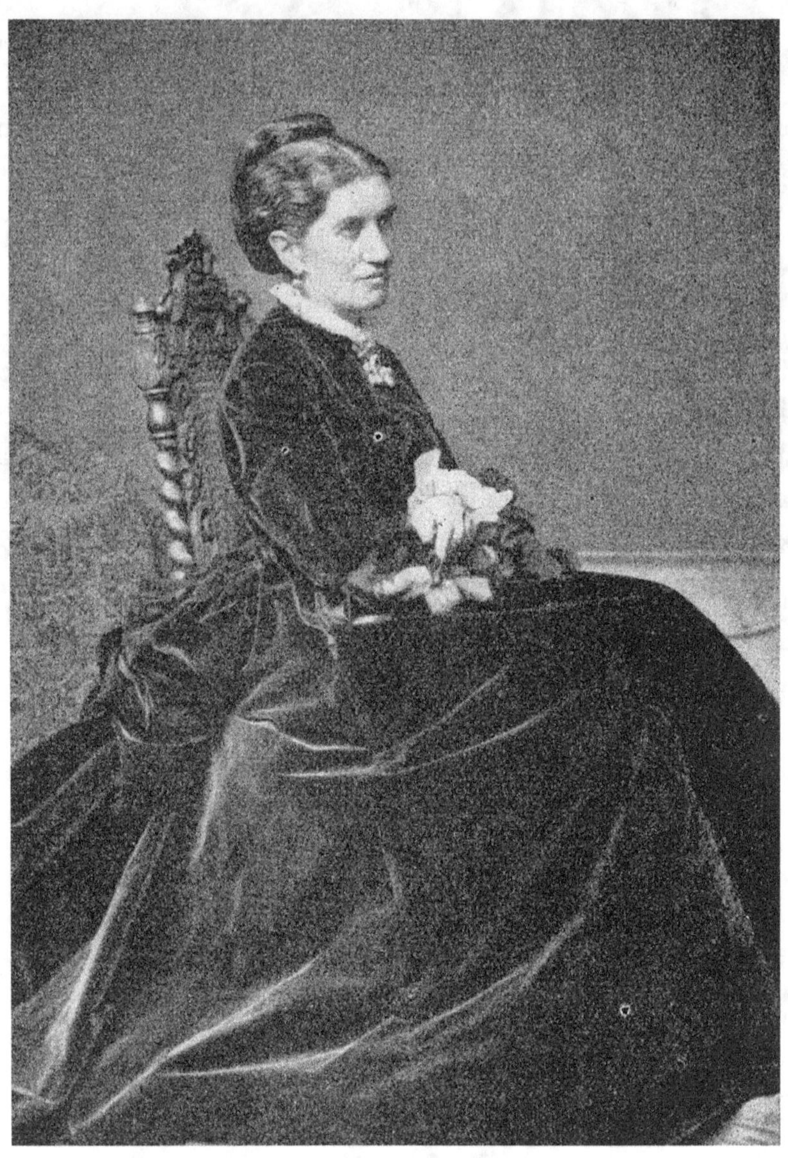

Johanna von Bismarck

In the Kingdom of Wurttemberg, one of the many states that constituted the federal German Empire, King Karl I (r. 1864–1891) and his wife Olga Nikolaevna of Russia both contracted the illness and suffered severely. On January 14, 1890, the renowned Roman Catholic theologian Johan Joseph Ignaz von Dollinger died from influenza at the age of 91. Dollinger had refused to accept the teaching of the First Vatican Council (1869–1870) on the infallibility of the pope in matters of dogma and morality and was subsequently excommunicated.

Influenza appeared in Vienna around the same time it reached Berlin. Vienna was the capital of the Austrian Empire, then in federation with the Kingdom of Hungary. The union was a curious entity among the community of European states as it was composed of several disparate ethnic populations, including Germans, Hungarians, Czechs, Serbs, Slovaks, Romanians, Poles, Ruthenians (Ukrainians), Croats, Slovenes and Italians. Austria-Hungary was not as industrialized as Germany, but in Western Europe it was second only to Germany in the extent of its railway network. It was bordered by mountains on every side, which would have slowed the spread of the influenza somewhat, but the River Danube and its heavy trade passed freely from Germany through both Vienna and Budapest.

When fears of influenza invading Austria first surfaced in mid-December 1889, two notable professors of the University of Vienna, Hermann Nothnagel and Otto Kahler, both pathologists, asserted that the disease was not contagious. Viruses would not be discovered and identified until 1898,[18] so they attributed the contagion to bacteria or even to that refuted but long-dying belief, *miasma*.[19] It was just a matter of days that the pestilence reached such levels in Vienna that the government ordered the closure of all the schools, and severe symptoms were reported in many patients.[20]

---

[18] Fenner F (2009). Mahy BW, Van Regenmortal MH (eds.). *Desk Encyclopedia of General Virology* (1 ed.). Oxford: Academic Press. p. 15.

[19] Kempińska-Mirosławska et alii.

[20] Ibid.

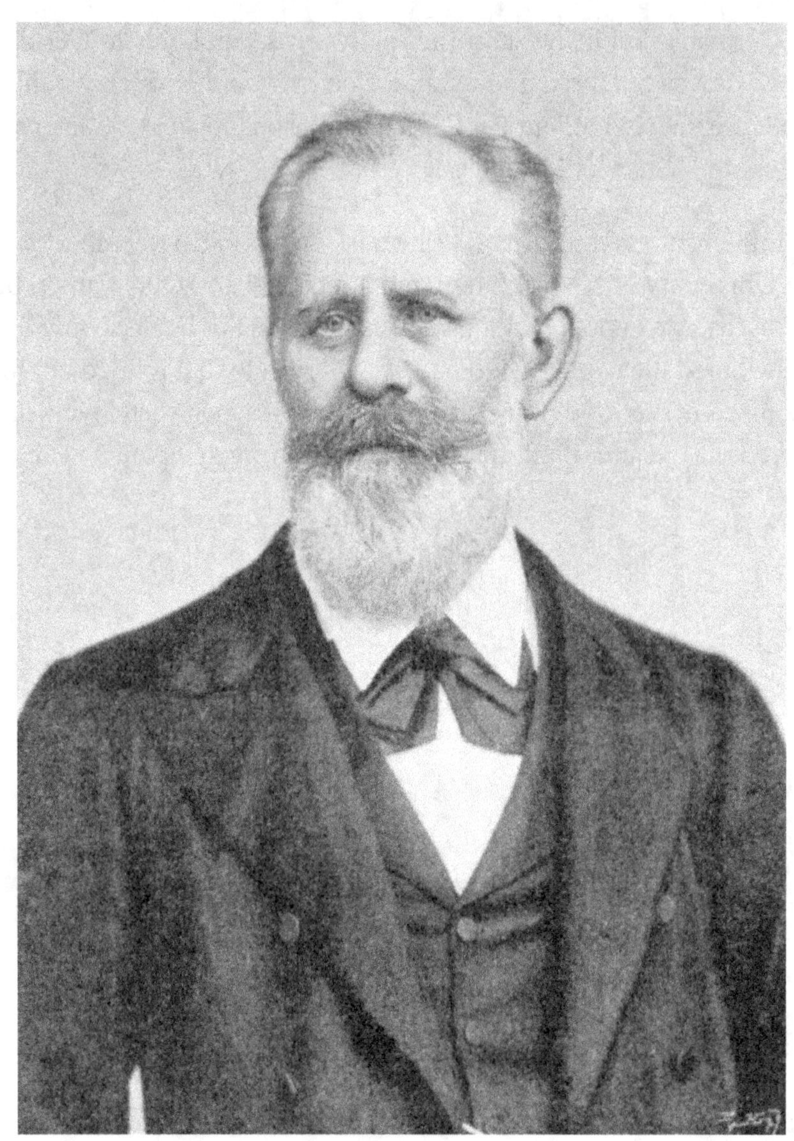

Nothnagel

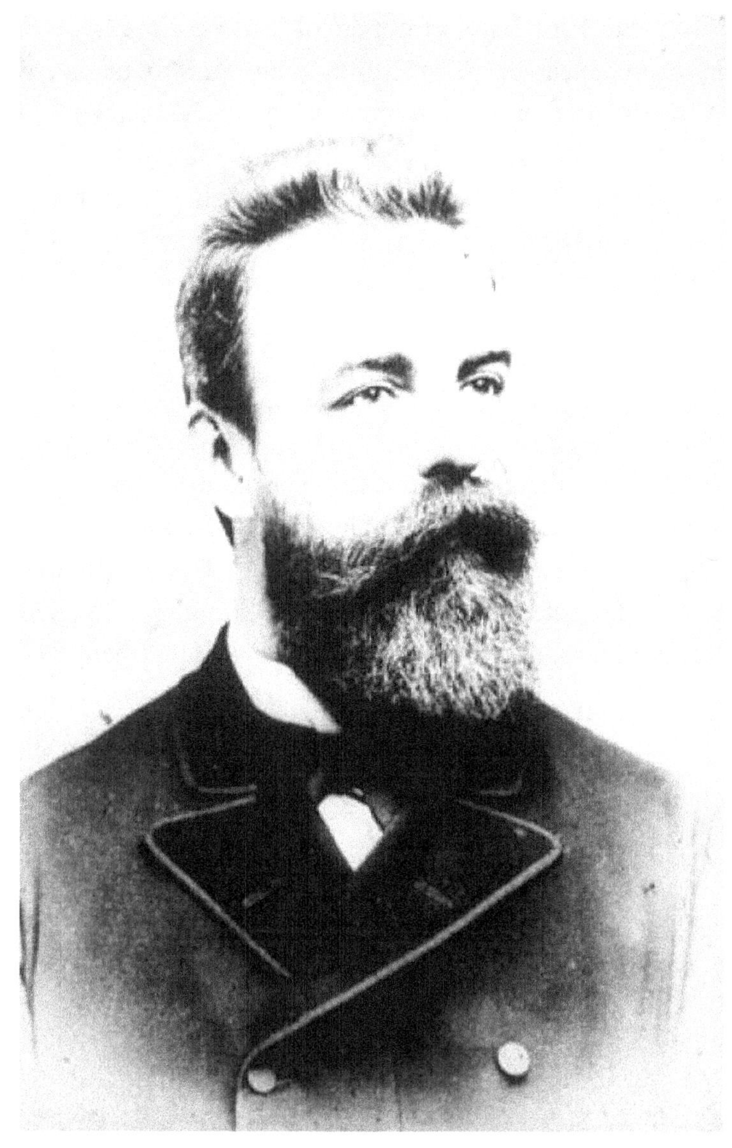

Kahler

Amongst the notable victims of the flu was Archduke Karl Ludwig (1833– 1896), the younger brother of the Emperor Franz Joseph I and father of the Archduke Franz Ferdinand, whose death precipitated the First World War in 1914. Archduke Karl Ludwig survived, only to die of another infectious disease – typhoid fever – seven years later.

In Vienna, the influenza only began to abate in late January 1891, and schools were reopened. At one point, one in three children were stricken, but none died. Four of the city's teachers were not so fortunate and succumbed to the disease.

By December 17, 1889 the influenza had reached Rome, reportedly brought by a group of Russian princes and their families.[21] Italy was a relatively new country thanks to its unification under Garibaldi in 1861, with King Victor Emmanuel II of Sardinia (r. 1849–1878) as its first king. Rome had been made the capital in 1871 after being forcibly taken from Pope Pius IX (r. 1846–1878), thus ending the thousand-year temporal rule of the bishops of Rome, and the unification of Italy was not universally welcomed by many inhabitants of former states that had existed for hundreds of years. Pius IX had proclaimed himself a "prisoner in the Vatican" in protest against the annexation of Rome, and he and his successor Leo XIII (r. 1878–1914) refused to recognize the legitimacy of the Italian state. Moreover, they forbade Catholics to do so as well, so there were pockets of armed resistance against what was widely deemed a Sardinian takeover, particular in southern Italy. Indeed, there was a great social and economic divide between the industrialized liberal north and the more rural and protectionist south.

This disparity meant that the epidemic would strike northern Italy first, but the south would suffer the most. A public health act, passed only in 1888, did something to alleviate the impact, and in the Vatican, Pope Leo XIII constructed Saint Mary's Hospice in preparation for an inundation of patients that did not ultimately come. In 1996, the refurbished building was set aside for papal conclaves, and today Pope Francis lives in an apartment there rather than in the Apostolic Palace.

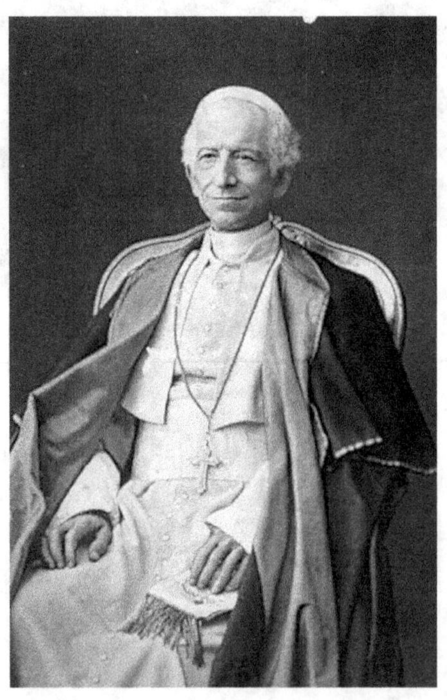

Pope Leo XIII

Prince Amadeo of Savoy was among the members of the Italian aristocracy affected by the epidemic. The second son of King Victor Emanuel II, the prince had already experienced an interesting if troubled career. In 1868, the liberal elite of Spain deposed Queen Isabella II and in

---

[21] Ibid.

August 1870 offered the vacant throne to Amadeo, but the unstable nature of Spanish politics ensured he was no more welcome than Isabella had been. There were uprisings against the government, and in 1872 he survived an assassination attempt. In February 1873 he appeared before the Cortes (Parliament) of Spain, declared the Spanish people ungovernable, and then returned to Italy, where he died of the flu on January 18, 1890. Tragically, his only son, Prince Umberto of Savoy, succumbed to influenza during the more notorious 1918 epidemic.

The epidemic reached France around the beginning of December 1889 and was first described by newspapers as a "mysterious disease" from St Petersburg.[22] As in many other countries, authorities attempted to strike a reassuring tone, highlighting the mildness of the symptoms in most individuals and expressing the opinion that precautions were unnecessary. However, by Christmas the hospitals were overcrowded, and hundreds died in Paris. Moreover, even as the scourge abated in the capital toward the end of December, it sprung up in other major regional centers, notably Grenoble, Toulon, Toulouse, Lyon, and Ajaccio (Corsica).

As that suggests, the flu spread quickly throughout the French Republic. Still smarting from defeat after the Franco-Prussian War (1870–1871), France was vigorously transforming its rural economy via a network of railways, seaports, and industries, all of which facilitated the epidemic. From the regional centers, the pestilence returned to Paris with a greater virulence than before. The Hôtel-Dieu, the oldest and most prestigious in Paris, reported that all its doctors had contracted the illness,[23] and in turn all the hospitals rapidly became overcrowded. Military barracks served as makeshift treatment stations and funeral directors were overwhelmed by demands, burying as many as 500 every day. Parisians were reminded of comparable casualties when Paris was under siege during the last nine weeks of the recent war – ultimately, 47,000 civilians died of famine and disease.

At the time the pestilence struck, France had just emerged from narrowly escaping civil war. After the war with Prussia, France was divided between the Revanchists, who wanted the return of the monarchy and revenge for the defeat and the loss of the border province of Alsace-Lorraine, and the more pragmatic Republicans represented by President Marie Francois Sadi Carnot (1837–1894). The Revanchists were led by Georges Boulanger (1837–1891), an officer of the French Army and a Minister of War until 1887 whose popularity was such that a coup seemed inevitable. He was indicted for treason and fled the country in April 1889, and his supporters contested the moderates in the general elections of July and were defeated. Boulanger shot himself in a Brussels cemetery two years later. After the elections, Carnot was recognized as the legitimate leader of France, so it was his government that the people turned to during the influenza epidemic. Carnot and several of his ministers fell ill but recovered.

---

[22] Ibid.
[23] Ibid.

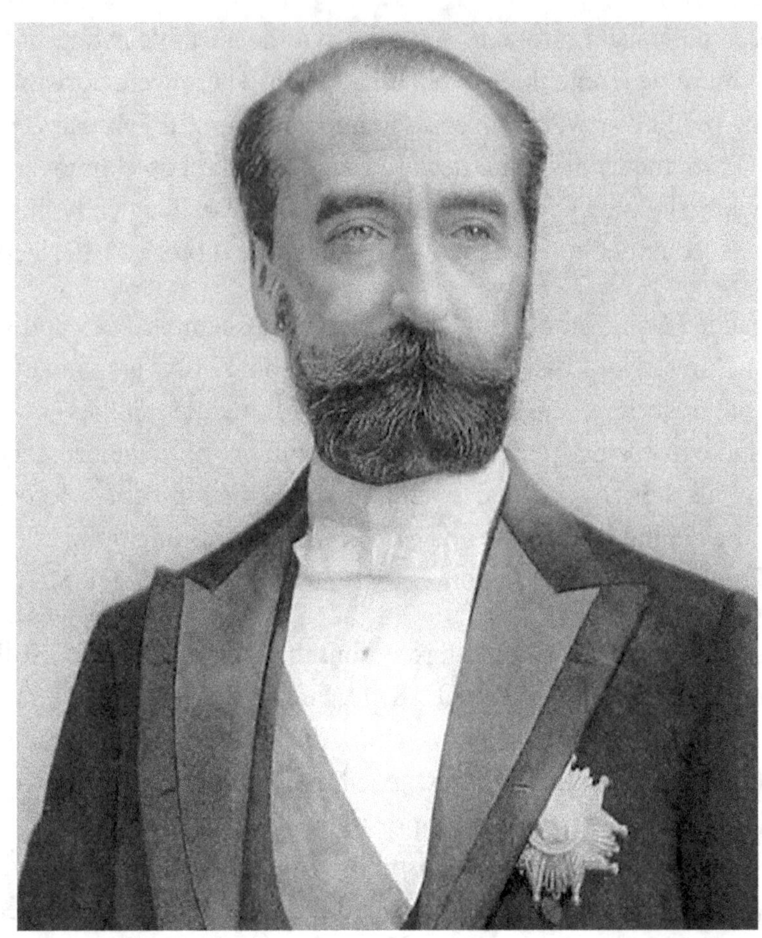

Carnot

The pestilence invaded the Kingdom of Spain toward the end of December 1889, appearing at a time when that unfortunate nation was in a state of turmoil. After its monarch Amadeo returned in disgust to Italy, Spain was proclaimed a republic for the first time, but the monarchy was restored in 1874 through Alphonso XII (r. 1874–1885), the son of Queen Isabella II. He died at the age of 28, leaving his son and heir still in the womb of Queen Marina Cristina of Austria (1858–1929), a member of the Austrian imperial family. The boy became Alphonso XIII upon his birth, and his mother took on the responsibilities of government on his behalf.

In 1889, the four-year-old king was described by the French newspaper *Le Figaro* as "the happiest and best-loved of all the rulers of the earth," but the influenza epidemic threatened to deprive the world of its joy. After contracting the disease, the young monarch seemed to rally, but his health deteriorated around January 10, 1890.[24] His doctors warned the regent, Maria Cristina, and her ministers to expect the worst. The queen's personal anxiety was dreadful, and the government feared that without a king the country would collapse into civil war again. To the relief of all, however, the little king rallied and continued to reign until his deposition in 1931.

---

[24] Ibid.

Beyond the royal palace of El Pardo in Madrid, the epidemic inflicted profound misery. By December 20, 20,000 inhabitants were ill, and a severe winter season added to the suffering of the people, with unemployed men, women, and children wandering the streets begging for food.[25] The state of public health in Spain was not advanced due to the unstable nature of its government, which left local governments responsible for providing sanitation and healthcare. A General Health Directorate had been established in 1855, but it only had the authority to coordinate the often poorly resourced local provincial governments.[26] In large cities like Madrid and Barcelona, three-quarters of those who contracted the disease developed pneumonia, in stark contrast with the situation in Germany and France. In Madrid, up to 300 people died each day and were buried at night so as not to panic the people.[27] Of course, such precautions were mostly futile since the misery was felt keenly by the Spanish people.

Being an island nation did not spare the United Kingdom, which should come as no surprise given its global reach. Its naval and merchant fleets, which made it the most powerful and prosperous nation on the planet, brought the plague to its shores. It arrived in London toward the end of December 1889 and at first seemed to show a preference for lawyers, rendering a number of courts silent for several days.[28] Postal clerks also bore a particularly heavy burden, but soon every class and occupation would be affected, including the aristocracy. Prime Minister Lord Salisbury (1830–1903) became ill but recovered well. Among the notables who succumbed was William Allen (1843–1890), a veteran of Rourke's Drift, an 1879 battle in the Anglo-Zulu War. His story was immortalized – somewhat inaccurately – in the 1964 film *Zulu*, which portrayed him as a model corporal in the 24th Infantry Regiment. In reality he had been demoted from the rank of sergeant for drunkenness on duty. In the eyes of his superiors he redeemed himself on January 22 and 23 of 1879 at Rorke's Drift by defending a military hospital and allowing the wounded to be withdrawn. He and Private Frederick Hitch were severely wounded, and after the patients were removed, they continued to assist by serving out ammunition to these beleaguered comrades. Both soldiers received the Victoria Cross for their actions. Allen died at his home in Monmouth on March 12, 1890 at the age of 46.

As in other nations, the disease rapidly spread to every other major city in the United Kingdom, particularly Birmingham, Glasgow, Edinburgh and Dublin.

While Europe was being ravaged, the citizens of the United States looked on with sympathy but not alarm. A pestilence originating in remote Russia could surely not reach their shores. Even

---

[25] Ibid.

[26] Sabino Cassese, Armin von Bogdandy, Peter Huber (eds), *The Max Planck Handbooks in European Public Law: Volume I: The Administrative State*, Oxford University Press 2017.

[27] Kempińska-Mirosławska et alii.

[28] Ibid.

when the first cases of influenza were reported in Boston on December 18, 1889, it caused no particular concern, which made sense since influenza was not an uncommon disease and an independent outbreak would not have been considered unusual. However, the disease spread along the East Coast and inland as far as Chicago and Kansas in a matter of days, even as journalists continued downplaying its significance. The *New York Evening World* reported, "It is not deadly, not even necessarily dangerous."[29]

On December 25, the first death in America occurred. Thomas Smith of Canton, Massachusetts was only 25 when he died, but by the first week of January 1890, over 1,200 Americans had died. Among the victims, all but 19 had chronic underlying conditions.

That same month, the pandemic reached San Francisco and other cities on the West Coast, and by the time the outbreak was done in America, just under 13,000 Americans had died, but not before it spread to Mexico and further south. By February 2, the disease had reached Buenos Aires.

Africa also succumbed to the depredations of the flu, which reached Port Natal in South Africa in November 1889. In February 1890, it had reached India, and by March the plague had spread to Singapore and the Dutch East Indies (modern Indonesia). By April it was in Japan, Australia, and New Zealand, and in May it tore through the Chinese Empire and returned to Central Asia, from where it had come less than a year earlier.

Thus, the grand network of railways, post offices, telegraphs, and merchant routes which made the powers of Europe and the Americas such dominant forces had carried contagion across the entire face of the globe in just one year. The 1889–1891 pandemic was the first of the modern pandemics in the sense that it was boosted by capitalism and industry, the very pillars of Western society.

As it turned out, the pestilence did not disappear in 1891. In fact, it would experience a resurgence across the world, not once, but four times.

The Resurgence

The pandemic of 1889–1890 was unique in human history in that it was the first time an outbreak of influenza had spread not just through Europe and Asia but to the entire world. This was possible because of railway networks, speedy sea and river routes, and national postal services, all undertakings of rapidly industrializing states. Ironically, even as those technological advances facilitated its spread, the identity of the influenza virus and the cause of the disease was unknown at the time, and the idea that infection was caused by microbiological organisms was still being debated. Many physicians still subscribed to the theory that contagion resided in foul

---

[29] Greg Daugherty, *The Russian Flu of 1889: The Deadly Pandemic Few Americans Took Seriously*, History.com March 23 2020 https://www.history.com/news/1889-russian-flu-pandemic-in-america.

or miasmic air derived from rotting organic matter. Just a few decades earlier, the eminent English physician and health reformer Thomas Wood (1788–1861) wrote, "To assume the method of propagation by touch, whether by the person or of infected articles, and to overlook that by the corruption of the air, is at once to increase the real danger, from exposure to noxious effluvia, and to divert attention from the true means of remedy and prevention."[30] Florence Nightingale, history's most famous nurse, concurred that germ theory excused physicians and health officials from action, operating under the mistaken belief that there could be no defense against invisible particles:

The idea of "contagion" as explaining the spread of disease grew at a time when the neglect of sanitary arrangements made it possible for epidemics to attack whole masses of people. In 1875, the German medical scientist Robert Koch successfully demonstrated that the bacterium *Bacillus antracis* was the cause of anthrax, a frightful condition that expresses itself in skin discoloration, lesions, fever, chills, coughing, chest pain, and shortness of breath. Practically speaking, however, the discovery – momentous as it was – was of no value if a vaccine could not be produced, and a vaccine for human anthrax was not available until 1954.[31] The bacterium for tuberculosis was identified – again by Koch – in 1882, but similarly, the discovery was of no practical benefit until there was a vaccine.

---

[30] "EBSCOhost Login". *search.ebscohost.com*. Archived from the original on 12 February 2018. Retrieved 7 May 2018.
[31] "Anthrax and Anthrax Vaccine – Epidemiology and Prevention of Vaccine-Preventable Diseases Archived 24 August 2012 at the Wayback Machine", National Immunization Program, Centers for Disease Control and Prevention, January 2006. (PPT format)

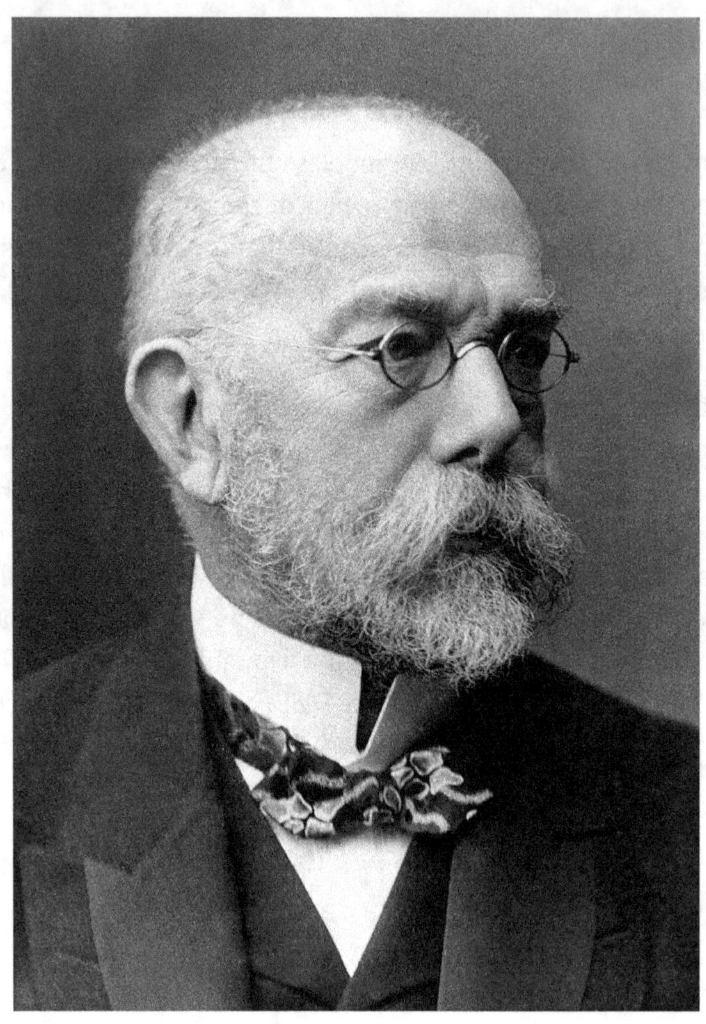

Koch

Physicians were divided on how to treat influenza in 1889 and in fact would remain divided during the Spanish Flu of 1918.[32] The drug quinine, most effective in the treatment of malaria, was frequently used in pill form as treatment but offered little benefit. The drug antipyrine (Phenazone) had been synthesized by the chemist Ludwig Knorr in 1887 and was prescribed as an analgesic, but it did nothing to aid recovery. Minute doses of strychnine were injected as stimulants, and doctors also prescribed liberal doses of whiskey and brandy, strong liquors that were often used for the relief of pain. For those who could not afford expensive drugs, there were plenty of traditional remedies that were prescribed, including poultices of ground linseed, salt and warm water, and glycerin (an antiviral agent) applied to the nostrils.

---

[32] Lisa Smith (February 6, 2018) "Nursing and Nutrition: Treating the Influenza in 1918–19", *The Recipes Report* https://recipes.hypotheses.org/10306.

Many people at the time adhered to the adage advising to starve a fever, which appears to have had its origin in a belief that food intake reduced the amount of heat the body produced. Fevers are indeed caused by the body burning calories, but this is a defensive mechanism of the body's immune system, so it's actually important to encourage a flu sufferer to eat in order to continue generating heat.[33]

Influenza was then, as now, a potentially lethal disease that typically led to mild symptoms for healthy people, but the young, old, and those with underlying conditions were the most vulnerable and often died of pneumonia or heart attack induced by physical stress. In the late 19th century, the numbers of vulnerable people were considerably higher than they would be today, owing to lower standards of living, worse hygiene, and the inability of medicine to treat chronic ailments that can be addressed today. This was true across the developed world, most notably Europe and America, so the effects on populations in sub-Saharan Africa and Asia were even more severe.

The pandemic resurged several times between 1891 and 1895, due in large to part to the medical uncertainty concerning the infectious nature of influenza and the inadequate measures taken to contain outbreaks. The first resurgence occurred as early as January 1891, and one of its first victims was the renowned and infamous Helena Blavatsky, a Russian émigré aristocrat who died in London on May 8, 1891. She had co-founded the Theosophical Society in the United States in 1875, and its founding members described the Society as "an unsectarian body of seekers after Truth, who endeavor to promote Brotherhood and strive to serve humanity."[34] They labored to "investigate the unexplained laws of nature and the powers latent in man" and in so doing made a study of occultism. After moving the headquarters to Madras (Chennai) in India, they proclaimed that mankind's destiny was being guided by a hierarchy of spiritual beings named the Masters of Ancient Wisdom. Unsurprisingly, Blavatsky claimed that the Theosophical Society, by which she meant herself, was the primary vehicle the spiritual beings used to speak and act in the real world. For Blavatsky and her disciples, all of creation was divine, moving inexorably toward a day of enlightenment and liberation from the darkness of Western religion.

Suffering from Bright's disease, Blavatsky headed to London in 1883 to strengthen the movement in the United Kingdom. She fled to Cairo a year later, after *The Times* published the claims of two former disciples, Emma and Ale Coulomb, that insisted she was a fraud. The Society for Psychical Research, an institution created in 1882 (and still exists) to scientifically examine claimed paranormal phenomena, sent Richard Hodgson to India to investigate Blavatsky's so-called spiritual and psychic powers. His report concluded that she was "one of the most accomplished, ingenious, and interesting impostors in history."[35] Hodgson accused

---

[33] Mark Fischetti (January 3, 2014) "Fact or Fiction?: Feed a Cold, Starve a Fever", *Scientific American* https://www.scientificamerican.com/article/fact-or-fiction-feed-a-cold/.

[34] *The Theosophical Movement 1875–1950*, Cunningham Press, Los Angeles 1951.

[35] Harrison, Vernon (1997). *H.P. Blavatsky and the SPR: an examination of the Hodgson report of 1885*. Pasadena, CA: Theosophical University Press.

Blavatsky of faking paranormal activity and moreover acting as a spy for the Russian government, which maintained interests in British India. The affair split the Society and greatly damaged its reputation, and Blavatsky was still fighting accusations of fraud when she died. Theosophists continue to commemorate her death as White Lotus Day.[36]

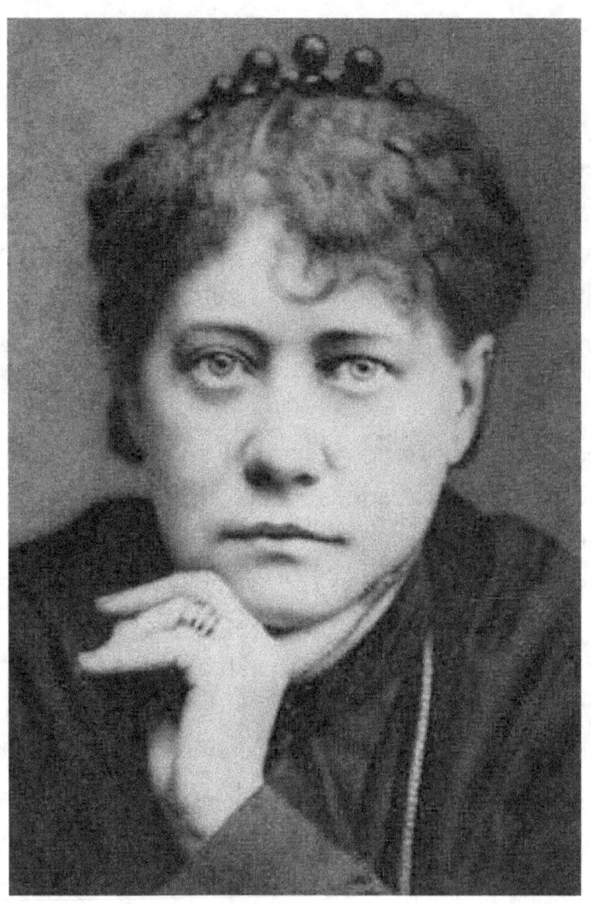

Blavatsky

Sofya Vasilyevna Kovalevskaya was another aristocratic woman who left her native Russia in pursuit of intellectual freedom. Born in 1850, she was the daughter of an officer in the imperial army with an extraordinary aptitude for mathematics, but she could not study mathematics in Russia, so she studied in Vienna, Heidelberg, and the prestigious University of Gottingen. Eventually, she achieved her doctorate and became the first woman in Europe to be awarded one, but when she returned to Russia in 1874, she found that her degree and considerable contributions to mathematical theory were unrecognized, and the political views of her putative husband Vladimir made them both social pariahs. After Vladimir's suicide, Sofya went to Sweden and secured a post as a lecturer at Stockholm University. In 1889, she was appointed the first female professor in Europe, even as her native Russia resolutely refused to offer her a

---

[36] <u>Lachman, Gary</u> (2012). *Madame Blavatsky: The Mother of Modern Spirituality*. New York: Jeremy P. Tarcher/Penguin, p.270.

professorship. She died in Sweden of influenza after vacationing in Nice on February 10, 1891. She was only 41.

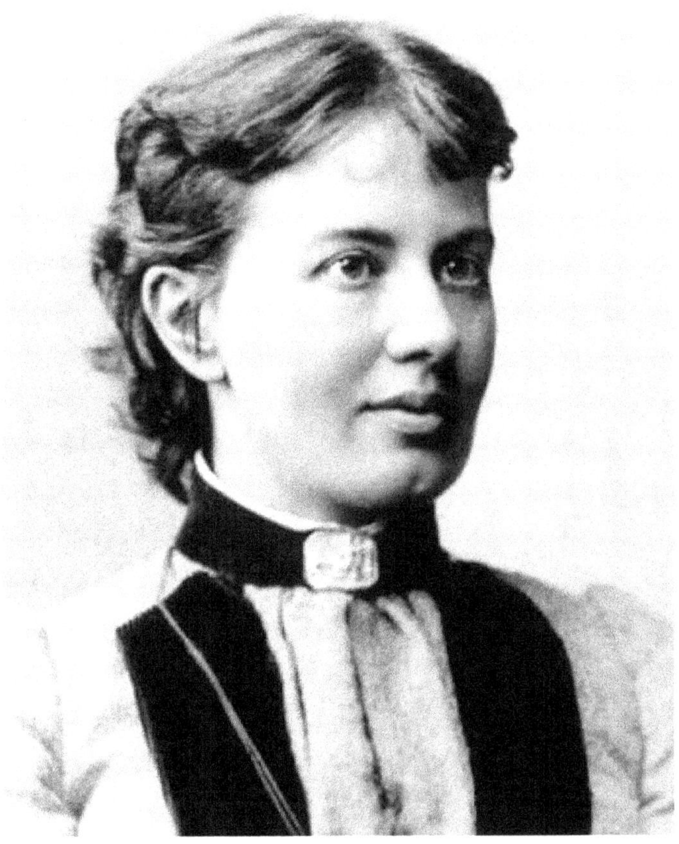

Kovalevskaya

In the United Kingdom another woman who broke barriers in her field was also struck down by the resurgence of the flu. Grisell Baillie, the first deaconess in the Church of Scotland, was the youngest of eleven children in a devoutly Presbyterian family. Her father was the Member of Parliament for Berwickshire and her mother was the daughter of a minor aristocrat. She devoted herself to philanthropic work and the temperance movement after giving up the vice of one small glass of wine with her dinner. When her brother George became the Earl of Haddington in 1858, she was entitled to the title of Lady, an honor which helped her in her charitable work. When in 1888 Archibald Charteris, a Church of Scotland minister and professor at the University of Edinburgh, instituted the office of deaconess, Lady Baillie became the first candidate. The Scottish Church has no bishops and is led by presbyters or elders. Until 1888 it did not have deacons, male or female, and in fact the diaconate was only opened to men in 1988.

Baillie was not the first woman in Europe to be appointed to the diaconate in modern times. The reformed Protestant movement had begun to admit women to the ministry in the 1830s, though churches took pains to state that women were not strictly ordained but appointed to assist the male ordained clergy. The commissioning of female deacons was not generally considered an equal rights issue, but the ministry gave women an opportunity for economic independence when the only respectable professions for them were teaching, nursing and domestic service. Lady Baillie died of the flu on December 20, 1891.

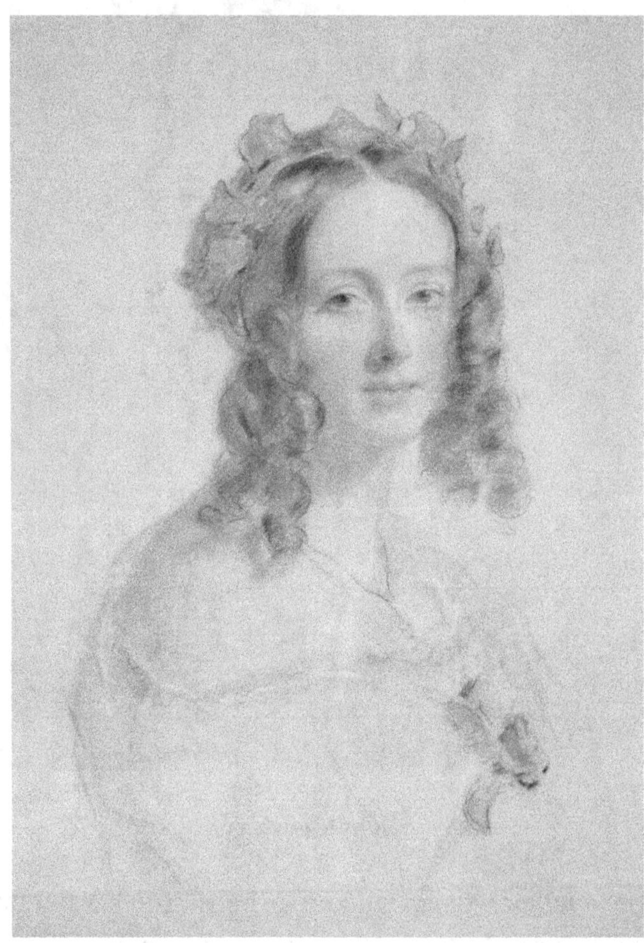

Lady Baillie

Eight days later another subject of Queen Victoria died in Berlin. Sir William Arthur White (b. 1824) was the son of Arthur White, a British diplomat, and Elizabeth Gardiner. Gardiner's father was the British Minister in Warsaw. After her father's death she remained in Poland, and Arthur was born in the town of Pulawy, Poland, which was then ruled by the Russian Empire. He followed in the careers of his father and maternal grandfather with distinction, accepting posts in Poland, Prussia, Serbia and Romania. His interventions in the Serbo-Bulgarian War of 1885 helped to ensure that the conflict did not escalate into a general European war. The situation in the Balkans remained an area of interest and expertise, and in 1886 he was appointed the United Kingdom's ambassador to the Ottoman Empire. The appointment generated some controversy, not on account of his undoubted credentials but because of his religion. He was raised a Roman Catholic, and although Roman Catholics had been allowed to enter the civil service since 1829, the cry "No popery" was still very strong in the United Kingdom. White was the first Roman Catholic to be appointed ambassador in Constantinople since the Protestant Reformation.

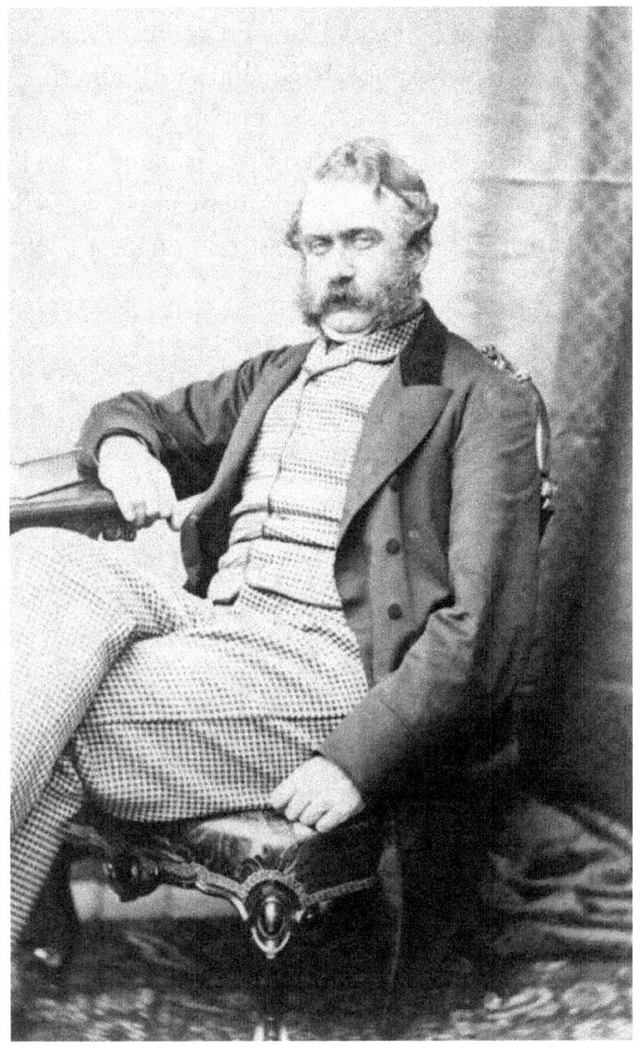

White

Sir William was unconventional in other regards as well. He married – in the estimation of many of his colleagues and peers – below his station. Katherine Marie Kendzior was the daughter of a German tobacconist, but White described his marriage to her as the greatest accomplishment of his career. She was graceful and powerful, but many could not accept that she should be the wife of an ambassador. One contemporary decried the fact that she visited the embassy kitchen and shopped for live turkeys in the markets of Constantinople.[37]

When Sir William died, he had recently been made a Knight of the Order of the Bath and a privy counselor. He was in Berlin at the time of his demise.

---

[37] McCarthy, Helen. *Women of the World: The Rise of the Female Diplomat*. New York: Bloomsbury, 2014. p. 45.

In 1892, a second epidemic broke out, and one of its first notable victims was Prince Albert Victor (b. 1864), the Duke of Clarence and Avondale and the eldest child of Edward Prince of Wales and Alexandra of Denmark. He was thus heir to the British throne after his father. He took after his father in pursuing a playboy's life, showing no interest or aptitude for education or public life. Nevertheless, his name was spoken frequently in 1889, after a male brothel was linked to members of the royal household and others in high society, including possibly the Duke of Clarence. The intervention of his father ensured that his name, if he had been involved, was never mentioned in court or the press. Undeterred, American media outlets, which had no sensitivity concerning the British Royal Family, referred to Albert Victor as a dullard and a perverse stupid boy.[38]

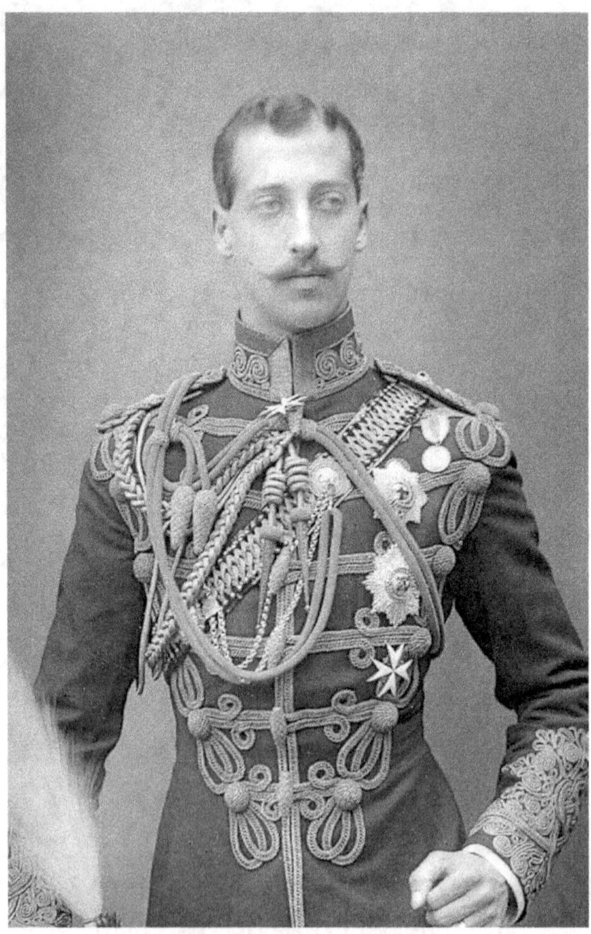

Prince Albert Victor

When Albert Victor set sail for a royal tour of India in 1889, his parents and grandmother (Queen Victoria) hoped that rumors about his private life would disappear, but controversy continued to dog him. A Mrs. Margery Haddon claimed that he was the father of her son, though

---

[38] Zanghellini, Aleardo (2015). *The Sexual Constitution of Political Authority: The 'Trials' of Same-Sex Desire*. Routledge. p. 150.

nothing was ever proven.

Marriage seemed the only cure for the prince's woes, and several prospective wives were lined up for him when he returned from India, but following a long tradition of royal children flouting their parents' wishes, he fell in love with Princess Helene of Orleans, a member of the exiled French Royal Family. The heir to the British throne could not by law marry a Roman Catholic, but the prince decreed that he would renounce the succession. To spare him this fate, Helene offered to convert to the Church of England. His father the Prince of Wales would have none of it and forbade the marriage outright, especially as it had been revealed that Pope Leo XIII had been approached by the princess for his consent.

Thwarted in love, the prince resumed his life of indulgence and debauchery. He had an affair with a chorus girl, Lydia Miller, who subsequently committed suicide by drinking carbolic acid. This time the newspapers of Britain did not spare the prince or his grandmother and parents. Victoria was adamant that her grandson settle down, and he was pressured into proposing to Princess Mary of Teck, the daughter of the queen's cousin, Princess Mary Adelaide of Teck. Plans were also under way to appoint him Viceroy of India, and it was hoped that marriage and responsibility might help the young man mature. Ultimately, it was not to be, as he suddenly fell ill, developed pneumonia, and died on January 14, 1892.

Though he was sincerely mourned by his family, the British press, and the nation, rumors and scandals pursued him even in death. In 1962, a journalist named Stephen Knight published a work in which he asserted that the notorious Jack the Ripper was none other than Albert Victor, the Duke of Clarence, a theory for which there is no evidence.[39]

Victor Albert's younger brother George replaced him in the line of succession, and George became king after his father Edward VII. George V married his elder brother's fiancée, and their eldest son became the infamous Edward VIII, who abdicated the British throne in 1936 and courted Nazis. His younger brother stepped in as George VI, just as his father had replaced his own brother in 1892, and George VI's daughter is none other than Queen Elizabeth II. In other words, it can be said that if there had not been an influenza pandemic in 1889, she would not be on the throne today.

1892 also brought the death of Amelia Edwards (b. 1831), the celebrated novelist, journalist, Egyptologist and traveler. She was born in London to a banker and his wife and showed promise as a writer from an early age. She published her first novel, *My Brother's Wife*, at the age of 24, and her novels were generally received warmly. She spent vast amounts of time researching them and included minute details in her works' settings and backgrounds, which may explain why she was such an ardent adventurer, exploring Europe often in the company of her friend

---

[39] . Cook, Andrew (2006). *Prince Eddy: The King Britain Never Had*. Stroud, Gloucestershire: Tempus Publishing Ltd, p. 8.

Lucy Renshawe, and often to the disdain of civilized society.

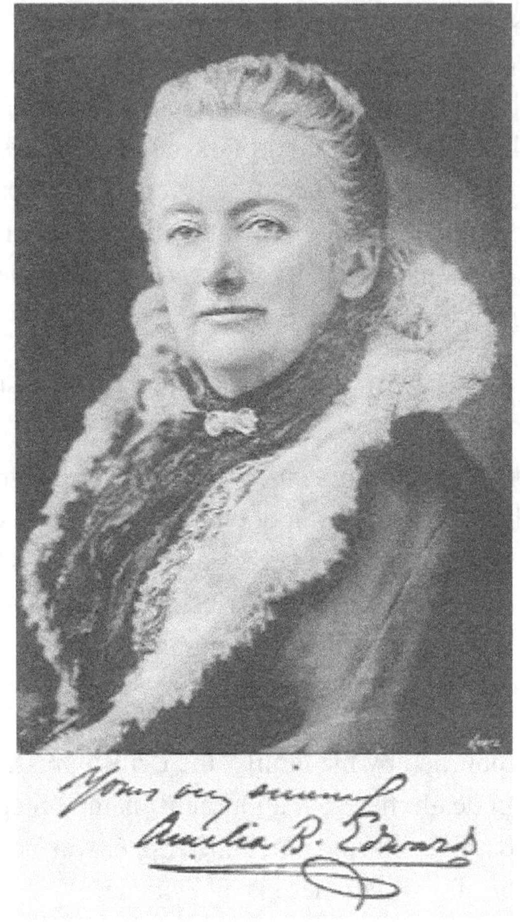

Edwards

In 1873, Edwards and Renshawe toured Egypt for the first time, and Edwards was instantly fascinated by the archaeological expeditions of men such as Flinders Petrie, whom Amelia was to meet in 1880. Her travelogues excited interest in ancient Egypt, and in 1882 she co-founded the Egypt Exploration Fund, a fundraising institution that exists to this day.

Amelia Edwards died on April 15, 1892 and was buried in the churchyard of St. Mary the Virgin Church in Bristol. She was laid to rest alongside her life partner of 30 years, Ellen Baysher, who died just three months before.

Across the English Channel, French naturalists were already mourning the passing of the biologist Jean Louis Armand de Quatrefages de Bréau (b. 1810). He was an exceedingly diligent, methodical academic who gained a number of prestigious positions in succession, including Professor of Natural History at the Lycee Napoleon, member of the French Academy of Sciences, Chair of Anthropology and Ethnography at the Museum National d'Histoire Naturelle and honorary member of the Royal Society of London, in addition to being made a Commander of the Legion of Honor. For all the honors and accolades heaped upon him in his own nation, he would not be particularly noteworthy had it not been for a couple of controversial theories.

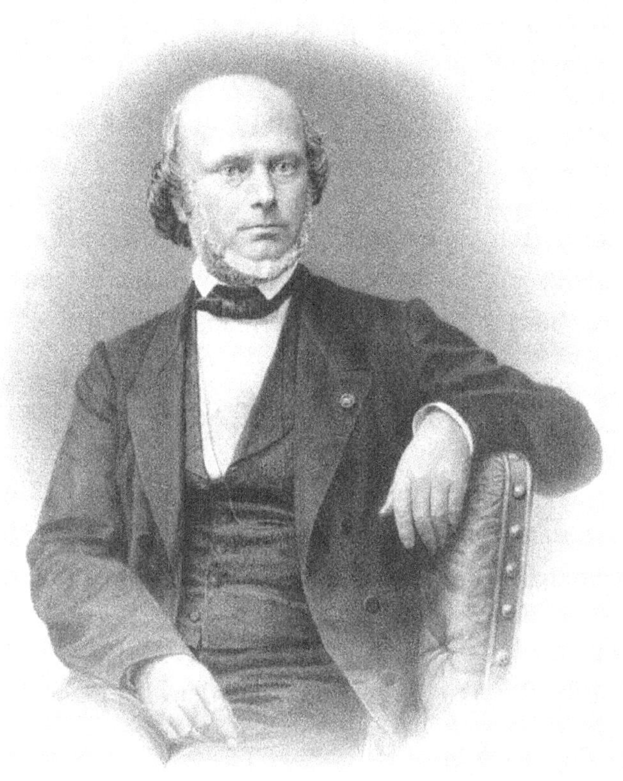

Jean Louis Armand de Quatrefages de Bréau

One of these theories, phlebenterism, proposed that in certain animals, organs can be replaced by others which retain the functions of the original organs. He claimed to have observed this in gastropods which he named *phelebenteres*, believing that they had once had circulatory systems, the functions of which were subsumed by the digestive tract. It was an obscure idea and has been completely debunked (gastropods do have a circulatory system but no blood vessels or even blood cells). Nevertheless, it generated little interest at the time and even more derision later.

Quatrefages de Bréau's advocacy of monogenism was also controversial at the time. This was the theory that all human races are derived from a single common ancestor. Monogenism is universally accepted today but in the 19th century the opposite opinion, polygenism, was almost universally held in scientific circles. The latter theory opined that the races of humanity were so different that they must have evolved independently. This conformed with the idea that some races were more advanced, more civilized, than others. The European peoples were naturally the highest, with the black-skinned peoples at the bottom and thus race segregation and colonial paternalism was justified on scientific grounds.[40] Within France, Quatrefages de Bréau was almost alone in his advocacy of monogenism, which was associated with Christianity and was thus unscientific. He was not, however, a creationist: he accepted the theory of evolution but not Charles Darwin's ideas as to how it worked. He did not believe that natural selection created new species, but rather that it would destroy them. He was quite forthright with Darwin but nevertheless remained friendly. The great English naturalist seemed not to have minded the criticism, writing to him "many of your strictures are severe enough, but all are given with perfect courtesy & fairness. I can truly say I would rather be criticized by you in this manner than praised by many others."[41] Quatrefages de Bréau died on January 12, 1892.

Thousands of miles from Europe, a Canadian inventor, Charles Fenerty, succumbed to influenza on June 10, 1892. For the contribution he has made to society, he is barely honored or even recognized. He was born the son of a lumberman and farmer in Nova Scotia and learned his father's trade, and he had a keen interest in wood processing and paper making in particular. When he was a teenager, paper was made from pulped rags, cotton and other plant fibers. This was a costly process and paper was still expensive, as it had been for hundreds of years. Nevertheless, there were increasing demands for paper during the 19th century, owing to the rapid rate of industrialization, literacy, and scientific progress. At the tender age of 17, Fenerty began his experiments in making paper from wood pulp, in consultation with the botanist Titus Smith (1768–1850).

In 1844, he triumphantly wrote to the Acadia Recorder on a piece of his newly manufactured paper:

> Messrs. English & Blackadar,
>
> Enclosed is a small piece of PAPER, the result of an experiment I have made, in order to ascertain if that useful article might not be manufactured from WOOD. The result has proved that opinion to be correct, for- by the sample which I have sent you, Gentlemen- you will perceive the feasibility of it. The enclosed, which is as firm in its texture as white, and to all appearance as durable as the common wrapping paper made from hemp, cotton, or the ordinary materials of manufacture is ACTUALLY COMPOSED OF SPRUCE WOOD, reduced to a pulp, and subjected to the same treatment as paper is in course of being made, only with this exception, VIZ: my insufficient means of giving it the required pressure. I entertain an opinion that our common forest trees, either hard or soft wood, but more especially the fir, spruce, or poplar, on account of the fibrous quality of their wood, might easily be reduced by a chafing machine, and manufactured into paper of the

---

[40] Hunt, James (24 February 1863). "Introductory address on the study of Anthropology". *The Anthropological Review*. **1**: 3.

[41] Burkhardt, Frederick. (2010). *Introduction*. In *The Correspondence of Charles Darwin: Volume 18; Volume 1870*. Cambridge University Press. pp. 21–22.

finest kind. This opinion, Sirs, I think the experiment will justify, and leaving it to
be prosecuted further by the scientific, or the curious.

I remain, Gentlemen, your obdt. servant,

CHARLES FENERTY.

The Acadian Recorder
Halifax, N.S.

Saturday, October 26, 1844[42]

Unfortunately, Fenerty never bothered to patent his invention, but some European inventors
did. Thus, he lost the opportunity to gain a place in history. The loss does not seem to have
embittered him, and he traveled the world extensively, taking a particular interest in Australia
during its gold rush period in the 1860s. He was also a poet of some note before he died at his
home in Lower Sackville, Nova Scotia.

---

[42] *Paper Maker and British Paper Trade Journal*. 1945. p. 363.

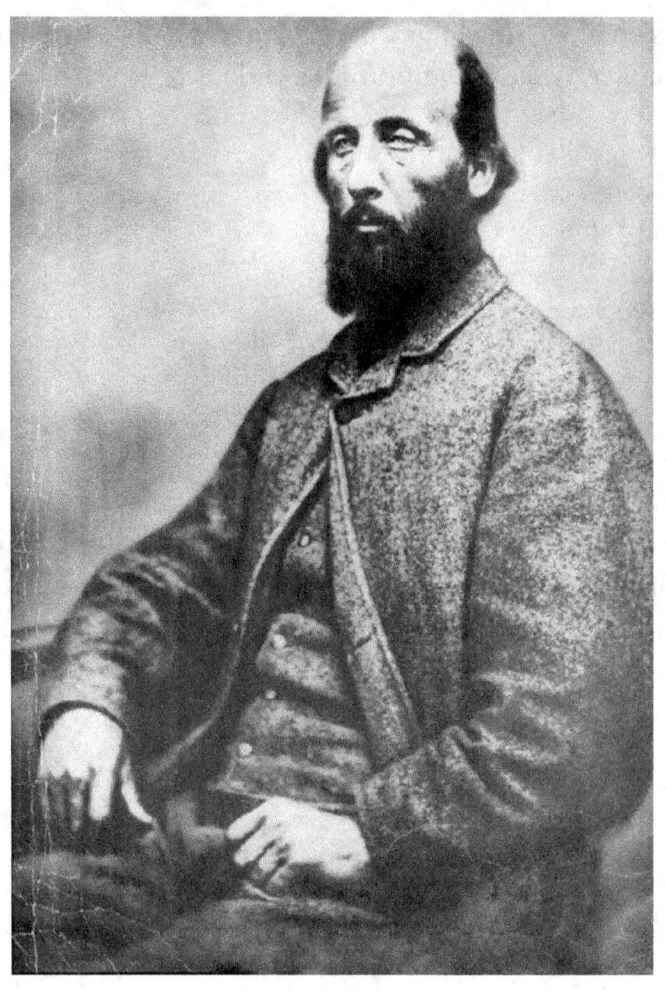

Fenerty

Further south in the United States, Gustavus Cheyney Doane lost his life on May 5, 1892. He had been a soldier and an explorer, but what limited fame he could claim was owed to his being one of the discoverers of the region of the western United States now known as Yellowstone National Park. In August 1870, he was selected by General Winfield Scott Hancock, a renowned veteran of the Civil War and the Mexican-American War, to lead a military escort for the Washburn Expedition. Lieutenant Doane was a skilled and resourceful leader, but it was his thorough and detailed observations that convinced Congress to create Yellowstone National Park on March 1, 1872, the first such park established in America.

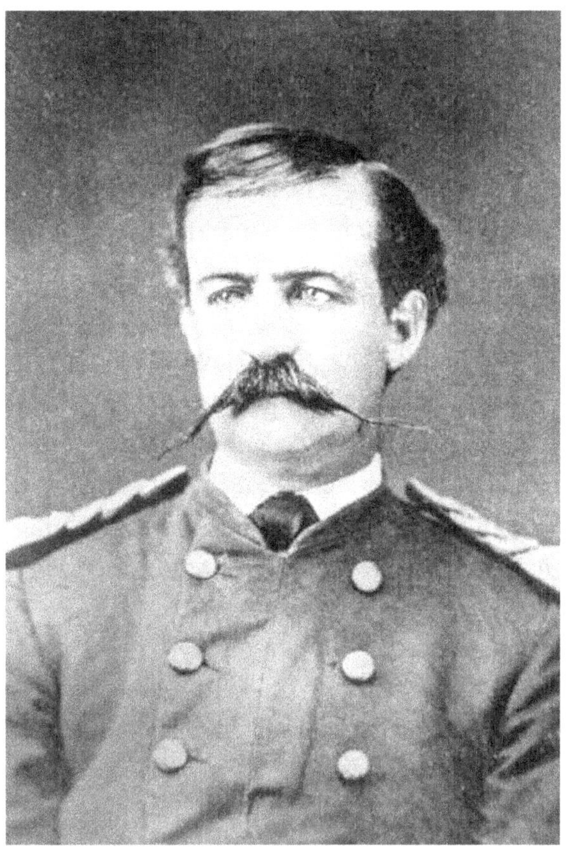

Doane

In an age when photography was still in its infancy, Doane's descriptions left members of Congress spellbound: "Along both banks of the Firehole River are the greatest of the geysers. Our camp was a few hundred yards below the first crater described, and the most beautiful of them all. Near the bank of the river, and a half a mile below camp, rose on the farther margin of a marshy lake the Castle Crater, the largest formation in the valley. The calcareous knoll on which it stands is 40 feet in height, and covers several acres. The crater is built up from its center, with irregular walls of spherical nodules, in forms of wondrous beauty, to a castellated turret, 40 feet in height and 200 feet in circumference at the base. The outer rim, at its summit, is formed in embrasures between large nodules of rock, of the tint of ashes of roses, and in the center is a crater three feet in diameter, bordered and lined with a frost-work of saffron. From a distance it strongly resembles an old feudal tower partially in ruins. This great crater is continually pouring forth steam, the condensation of which keeps the outside walls constantly wet and dripping."[43]

The mission to Yellowstone and the accolades he received gave Doane a taste for exploration. Inspired by explorers like Dr. Livingstone and Henry Morton Stanley, he pressed the War Department to send him on an expedition to survey the Nile. This was refused, though the

---

[43] Doane, Gustavus C., Lt. U.S. Army (February 1871). The report of Lieutenant Gustavus C. Doane upon the so-called Yellowstone Expedition of 1870 (Report). U.S. Secretary of War.

Secretary of War did send him back to Yellowstone. In 1876 he obtained permission to lead an expedition along the Snake River, south of Yellowstone, but he was recalled without completing the survey after endangering the lives of his team in pursuit of his own personal ambition.

In 1880, Doane, still hungry for adventure, obtained the army's permission to accompany Captain Henry Howgate on an expedition to Greenland. The US Army withdrew its support when it discovered that the steamship *Gulnare* was unfit for this purpose. This did not prevent Howgate and Doane from seeking private funding. The expedition failed because the *Gulnare*, captained by Doane, was forced to turn back in the face of a heavy gale. Nevertheless, Doane claimed it as a triumph of sorts in that 'We did not change the names of all the localities visited, as is customary, nor give them new latitudes to the bewilderment of the general reader. We do not dispute anyone's attained distance nor declare it impossible that he should have been where he was. We did not hunt up nameless islands and promontories to tag them with the surnames ... We did not even erect cenotaphs ... We received no flags, converted no natives, killed no one ...'[44]

After these events Doane was promoted to the rank of captain and given assignments in the Indian wars, during which he recovered the remains of Colonel George Armstrong Custer from the field of Little Big Horn. He retained an interest in Yellowstone and was deeply disappointed that he was passed over for the post of military superintendent of the park. He died in retirement in his hometown of Bozeman, Gallatin Valley County, Montana.

Influenza broke out again in 1893 and 1894. In 1894, one of the victims was John Thompson Ford (b. 1829), who was famous in his time as the proprietor of the theater named after him, Ford's Theatre. Ford's Theatre was where President Abraham Lincoln was shot by John Wilkes Booth on April 14, 1865. Ford was successful and well-known in his own right before the assassination as a playwright and manager of a number of theaters. He was also President of the City Council of Baltimore in 1858 and acting mayor for two years.

Unfortunately, Ford was good friends with Booth, who was an actor of considerable renown, and it did not help his reputation that he was in Richmond, the recently occupied capital of the Confederacy, when Lincoln was murdered. On April 18, 1865, Ford was arrested along with his brothers Harry and James, only to be released 39 days later for lack of evidence. To add insult to injury, his theater was forcibly purchased by the government for $88,000. Though he remained bitter on account of his treatment and loss of reputation, he did recover, and when the Gilbert and Sullivan operetta craze swept America in the 1870s, he was the only manager licensed to produce their plays in the United States because he was known to be scrupulously honest. He died of an influenza-induced heart attack at his Baltimore home on March 14, 1894.

The year 1895 saw yet another global outbreak of influenza and the deaths of several eminent

---

[44] "Polar sarcasm, Lieut. Doane, of the Howgate expedition, presents an ironic report" (PDF). *pdf*. The New York Times. 1881-04-11.

and interesting individuals. One of these was John Hulke, a British surgeon and geologist who grew up in Kent. He served in the Crimean War (1853–56) and was appointed assistant-surgeon at the Siege of Sebastopol, an exceedingly bloody affair that brought the deaths of over 138,000 British, French, and Italian troops. He worked alongside Florence Nightingale, struggling with the appalling conditions of military medicine at the time, and after the war he established a noteworthy career as a surgeon in England, where he specialized in ophthalmology.

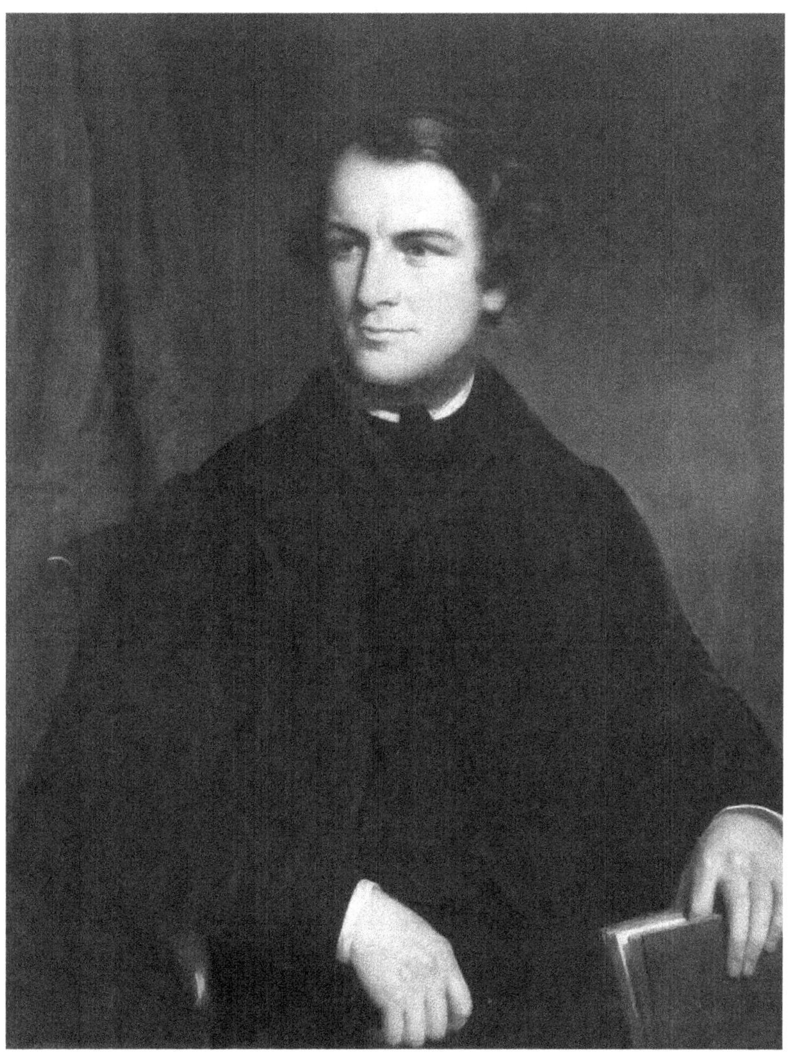

Hulke

Unlike Nightingale, he didn't resolve to spend every waking hour working to reform British healthcare. Rather, his passions leaned in an entirely different direction. Collecting fossils was a favorite pastime of many wealthy gentlemen who were excited by recent descriptions of giant reptilian bones by men like William Buckland (1784–1856), Gideon Mantell (1790–1852) and Richard Owen (1804–1892). Owen was Britain's foremost anatomist and natural historian and had proclaimed the existence of a new group of extinct reptiles which he called the *Dinosauria*. Dinosaur-mania had hit the world, and Dr John Hulke was one of the most prominent enthusiasts. He spent many of his spare hours on the Isle of Wight, where the remains of dinosaurs and other prehistoric creatures had been found. He overcame his strict Calvinist views to consider the possibility that a fantastical and humanless world existed before the Biblical flood, and his research uncovered an ancient tropical world in England when the Isle was joined to the mainland. He was the first to give a detailed description of the strange dinosaur *Polacanthus,* which sported thick bony spikes on its back and flat vertical plates along its tail. He reconstructed the first small herbivorous dinosaur known to science, *Hypsilophodon*, imagining it to be a lizard-like creature that scampered up trees for protection. Today paleontologists regard the dinosaur as a fleet biped. He also discovered several species of large long-necked herbivores called sauropods. These are little known to the public, with decidedly uncatchy names such *Eucamerotus, Ornithopsis, Ceteosaurus and Ischyrosaurus.* Hulke also uncovered the remains of a large plated dinosaur similar to that named *Stegosaurus* in the United States. He named his version *Omosaurus durobrivensis.*

   The ancient fossilized realms did not, however, distract him from medical interests, or from receiving accolades in the Geological Society. He earned the praises of the medical profession when he was made President of the Royal College of Surgeons in 1893, and he was about to deliver the Hunterian Oration, an annual lecture, to the College when he died of influenza on February 19, 1895.

   Unlike most others killed by influenza, Joseph Thompson was young when he died on February 14, 1895 at the age of 37. Like Hulke, he was a geologist, but his interest did not lead him to examine ancient bones, as he relished the thrill of discovery as an explorer. The vast African continent below the Sahara was mostly unknown to Europeans, and Thompson eagerly joined an expedition of the Royal Geographical Society in 1878 as its geologist. It was his first assignment after graduating from the University of Edinburgh. The goal of the expedition was to chart a route from Dar es Salaam in Tanzania to Lake Tanganyika. Five years later he accompanied the Society again, this time to establish a route from eastern Africa to Lake Victoria. His enthusiasm, observations and leadership skills earned him renown, and his adventures inspired many back in the United Kingdom, including the writer Henry Rider Haggard, who wrote *King Solomon's Mines* after hearing an account of Thompson's adventures.

The Aftermath

   The connection of the entire world via communication networks in the latter half of the 19th century rendered the globe vulnerable to a multitude of infectious diseases at a time when infection was still little understood. The bacteria and viruses that caused these diseases were still being identified, and serious scientists and physicians were still talking about miasmic air at the turn of the century, but germ theory was beginning to dominate the medical schools and hospitals of Europe and America, and emphasis was being put on personal hygiene, sanitation, and drinking clean water. Unfortunately, vaccines for most of the contagious diseases, such as mumps, measles, chickenpox, meningitis, polio, and influenza, were not developed until the latter half of the 20th century. Antibiotics, which are only effective against bacteria, were not widely available until the 1940s, and antiviral drugs were only developed in the 1960s (even now, antiviral drugs are not generally used for influenza).

Thus, despite enormous advances in medical science, successful remedies against most contagious illnesses were still not on the horizon, and an even worse influenza pandemic struck the globe in 1918. Aside from the Black Death during the Middle Ages, the Spanish Flu may be the most notorious outbreak in history, and it claimed up to 50 million lives. That strain of flu was particularly severe, and though it killed predominantly sick and elderly people, it also took the lives of young adults disproportionately compared to seasonal flu outbreaks. The Spanish Flu also resurged twice, much the way the flu of 1889 resurged and devastated many communities. In fact, the second and third outbreaks, which occurred in 1919, were more lethal than the first. The economic effects of the Spanish Flu were devastating, as stores were closed on account of quarantine or lack of manpower, and in many places the sick could not be attended to for lack of able-bodied health workers. Graves could not be dug for the same reason. Many who survived also suffered through the loss of livelihoods, a shortage of goods and services, and social isolation and poverty, a situation not unfamiliar to those suffering from the response to the COVID-19 pandemic.

To date, the Spanish Flu has been the worst flu pandemic, but it was not the last one. There have since been three more. The 1957–58 pandemic may have caused four million deaths, as did the pandemic of 1968–69, four times the number inflicted by the 1889 pandemic. The 2009 influenza pandemic, also known as the swine flu pandemic (though it was not carried by pigs), may have caused up to 575,000 deaths, significantly less than those caused by seasonal flu, which is up to 650,000 per year.[45] Swine flu was worse than seasonal flu in that it was unusually severe for young adults.

Many around the world to this day don't realize that seasonal flu is so lethal. Each year it infects millions around the world and kills hundreds of thousands of people, making it one of the world's biggest causes of death. Indeed, it will probably continue to be so for the foreseeable future. Medical scientists constantly research pharmaceuticals and vaccines that may provide some surer protection from future pandemics, but the difficulty lies in the fact that the influenza virus is capable of rapid mutation and evolution into new strains, which is why new flu vaccinations are put on the market each year. There is at present no universal influenza vaccination that could be effective against every strain, despite the fact attempts have been made to produce one.[46]

---

[45] "Up to 650,000 people die of respiratory diseases linked to seasonal flu each year". *World Health Organization (WHO)* (Press release). 14 December 2017.

[46] Nachbagauer R, Krammer F (April 2017). "Universal influenza virus vaccines and therapeutic antibodies". *Clinical Microbiology and Infection*. **23** (4): 222–228.

Some antiviral medications can be used in the treatment of influenza, but all they do is reduce symptoms.[47] The best measures against influenza remain preventative, such as maintaining good personal health and hygiene, public sanitation, staying home when sick, and avoiding contact with sick people.

The discussion of past pandemics naturally leads to the present COVID-19 pandemic, but it is not a form of influenza. Rather, it is a form of Coronavirus, belonging to the same group of viruses as some strains of the common cold. Some of the symptoms of COVID-19 are similar to influenza, including fever, coughing, sore throat, and muscle pains, and as with influenza, it can progress to pneumonia and other life-threatening conditions.[48] To date, there is no vaccine for COVID-19 and no effective tested treatment.

Periodic pandemics such as those of COVID-19 and influenza highlight the vulnerability of the modern world to infectious diseases, and in some ways the world is even more vulnerable than in 1889. In that year, newly-constructed railway networks facilitated the spread of disease, but the 21st century has air travel, faster trains, an increased volume of fast personal vehicles, increased shipping and commercial transportation productivity, and other ways for potentially lethal microorganisms to swiftly travel and infect communities.

This has not gone unnoticed by public health experts. On September 10, 2018, a new international body calling itself the Global Preparedness Monitoring Board [49] convened to "monitor progress, identify gaps and advocate for sustained, effective work to ensure global preparedness."[50] Its first annual report, titled *A World at Risk*, warned that the world was completely unprepared for "a very real threat of a rapidly moving, highly lethal pandemic of a respiratory pathogen killing 50 to 80 million people."[51] The organization was assembled by the World Health Organization and the World Bank and made this prediction without any direct

---

[47] Ebell MH, Call M, Shinholser J (April 2013). "Effectiveness of oseltamivir in adults: a meta-analysis of published and unpublished clinical trials". *Family Practice*. **30** (2): 125–33.

[48] Mehta, Puja; McAuley, Daniel F.; Brown, Michael; Sanchez, Emilie; Tattersall, Rachel S.; Manson, Jessica J. (28 March 2020). "COVID-19: consider cytokine storm syndromes and immunosuppression". *The Lancet*. **395** (10229): 1033–1034.

[49] World Health Organization (September 10, 2018) "Global Preparedness Monitoring Board convenes for the first time in Geneva" https://www.who.int/news-room/detail/10-09-2018-global-preparedness-monitoring-board-convenes-for-the-first-time-in-geneva.

[50] Ibid.

[51] GMBD Annual Report 2019, as quoted by Sigal Samuel (September 19, 2019) "The next global pandemic could kill millions of us. Experts say we're really not prepared." *Vox* https://www.vox.com/future-perfect/2019/9/19/20872366/global-pandemic-prevention-who-world-bank-report.

foresight of the calamitous events that would rapidly unfold within a matter of months. The warning was largely ignored, and even when the first cases of COVID-19 in China were reported by WHO, most governments were large unconcerned.[52]

In 1889, the initial reaction of governments and the press was to ignore, or to at least downplay the significance of outbreaks of influenza. In some cases, this was done to avoid panic, but in general there seemed to have been a feeling that a pandemic, if it did occur, would have minimal impact. When faced with danger, people often panic or else deny the danger, so in general there was little preparation for the influenza outbreak in 1889. Europe and America were still coming to terms with the impact of rapid and civilization-changing technological advances, and perhaps its inhabitants honestly did not expect that these very advances would allow the pestilence to move so quickly.

Either way, there have been attempts to establish international cooperation regarding pandemics since the 19th century, and some of them predated the 1889 pandemic. In 1834, a French health administrator called for an international body to establish common standards, in particular to overcome "disastrous hindrances to international commerce' occasioned by pandemics."[53] Such a body, called the International Sanitary Conference, did come into being, but it only met 14 times between 1851 and 1938, as it suffered from medical and political disagreements. It was not until 1926, the group's penultimate meeting, that nations agreed to notify each other of the first confirmed cases of infectious diseases such as bubonic plague, cholera, yellow fever and typhus. Somewhat perversely, it did not categorize influenza as a notable threat because it was deemed practically impossible to quarantine it.[54]

During World War I and World War II, international cooperation regarding health and sanitation was virtually nonexistent, but with the establishment of the United Nations came the World Health Organization, which began functioning in 1948. In 1969, UN member states agreed to report outbreaks of contagion to WHO, which monitors them and provides warnings and guidelines to states concerning epidemics and pandemics, including influenza. However, international health regulations are only effective if member states observe them in good faith, and in the case of COVID-19, the international response has been varied, with China not being forthright about the nature of the virus with the WHO and some countries virtually ignoring the initial warnings. The recent rise of nationalism and decline of globalism may compound the problem of formulating an internationally coordinated response to the latest pandemic, so infectious diseases such as influenza and COVID-19 will almost certainly continue to threaten the world, all while deadly diseases hitherto unknown to scientists may burst onto the scene and

---

[52] Alec Padua, "WHO warned the world as early as January in response to US', *Micky* April 17, 2020
   https://micky.com.au/who-warned-the-world-as-early-as-january-in-response-to-u-s/.
[53] Norman Howard Jones, Scientific Background of the International Sanitary Conferences 1851–1938, History
   International Public Health 1 (1975).
   p.11, https://apps.who.int/iris/bitstream/handle/10665/62873/14549_eng.pdf
[54] Jones, p. 97.

challenge humanity.

Online Resources

<u>Other books about the plague on Amazon</u>

Free Books by Charles River Editors

We have brand new titles available for free most days of the week. To see which of our titles are currently free, <u>click on this link</u>.

Discounted Books by Charles River Editors

We have titles at a discount price of just 99 cents everyday. To see which of our titles are currently 99 cents, click on this link.

www.ingramcontent.com/pod-product-compliance
Lightning Source LLC
Chambersburg PA
CBHW060522120726
48002CB00011B/3277